The Coconut Oil & Low-Carb Solution

For Alzheimer's, Parkinson's, and Other Diseases

A STEP-BY-STEP GUIDE TO USING DIET AND HIGH-ENERGY FOODS TO PROTECT AND NOURISH THE BRAIN

MARY T. NEWPORT, M.D.

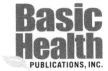

Basic Health PUBLICATIONS, INC.

The information contained in this book is based upon the research and personal and professional experiences of the author. It is not intended as a substitute for consulting with your physician or other healthcare provider. Any attempt to diagnose and treat an illness should be done under the direction of a healthcare professional.

The publisher does not advocate the use of any particular healthcare protocol but believes the information in this book should be available to the public. The publisher and author are not responsible for any adverse effects or consequences resulting from the use of the suggestions, preparations, or procedures discussed in this book. Should the reader have any questions concerning the appropriateness of any procedures or preparation mentioned, the author and the publisher strongly suggest consulting a professional healthcare advisor.

Basic Health Publications, Inc.

www.basichealthpub.com

Library of Congress Cataloging-in-Publication Data

Newport, Mary T.
 The coconut oil and low-carb solution for Alzheimer's, Parkinson's, and other diseases / Mary T. Newport, M.D.
  pages cm
 Includes bibliographical references and index.
 ISBN 978-1-59120-381-0 (Pbk.)
 ISBN 978-1-68162-909-4 (Hardcover)

1. Alzheimer's disease—Diet therapy. 2. Coconut oil—Therapeutic use. 3. Fatty acids—Therapeutic use. I. Title.
 RC523.N536 2015
 616.8'310654--dc23

              2015024162

Editor: Cheryl Hirsch
Typesetting/Book design: Gary A. Rosenberg
Text illustrations: Joanna Newport
Cover photos: Kathryn O'Malley
Cover design: Kimberly Richey

Contents

PART THREE

The Science

Appendices

"There's no place like home."
—DOROTHY, *THE WIZARD OF OZ*

This book is dedicated to Steve, the love of my life,
who made it possible for me to be both mother and doctor.
He may ultimately lose his battle with Alzheimer's,
but we are fighting it together with everything we have.
Hopefully, the path we have taken in our battle
will make it possible for many others to win.

This book is also dedicated to our helpers
who have endured the unimaginable—
true friends and true caregivers who fight this battle with us
and make it possible to keep Steve at home with me.

Acknowledgments

Like my previous book, this one would not exist were it not for the dedication and persistence of Richard L. Veech, M.D., Ph.D., who, over many years, has pursued what ketones do and how they might be used as an alternative fuel to make lives better for people with Alzheimer's, Parkinson's, amyotrophic lateral sclerosis, multiple sclerosis, and a myriad of other conditions. There are not enough words to express how sincerely grateful we are for what he has done to give our family extra quality years with my husband and our children's father, Steve. I also wish to thank M. Todd King, Yoshira Kashiwaya, M.D., and the many others who have worked alongside Dr. Veech in the pursuit of knowledge about ketones.

I also wish to acknowledge Theodore B. VanItallie, M.D., for his mentorship and his tireless efforts in getting information about ketones as an alternative fuel out to the scientific community.

I want to express my deepest appreciation to our helpers, who have made it possible for us to provide Steve with "assisted living" at home for nearly three years now, surrounded by people who truly love and care for him, our daughter Joanna Newport, her husband Forrest Rand, and other caregivers Sybil Kennedy, Joseph Brust, and Nemuel Major. Without them, taking care of Steve at home would be truly impossible. I also wish to thank Joanna for her graphic designs and her help with keeping up my website and Facebook pages. I also want to recognize the love and support of our daughter Julie DiPalo, and our many other family members and friends.

I wish to express my love and deepest appreciation to my sister Angela Bertke for always being there for me and for her never-ending moral support. I also want to thank her for the many hours spent critiquing and proofreading this book, as well as getting the message out to others. I want to thank her husband John Bertke, my brother-in-law, for caring and being right there behind her.

I want to recognize Dominic D'Agostino, Ph.D., at the University of South Florida, for his friendship, moral support, and dedication to researching how ketones might benefit children and adults suffering from epilepsy, cancer, and neurodegenerative diseases, and for otherwise spreading the "gospel of ketones." I also wish to thank David Morgan, Ph.D., of the Byrd Alzheimer's Institute at the University of South Florida for recognizing the potential of ketones as a treatment and for conducting the first pilot study of coconut oil in people with Alzheimer's that I am aware of.

I want to acknowledge the publisher Norman Goldfind for putting this message into print, editor Cheryl Hirsch for her expertise and guidance, and publicist Courtney Dunham for her great help in bringing this message to the public.

Most important, I want to thank my husband, Steve, for more than forty years of love, support, and patience and for being the kind of person you want to fight for.

Preface

"One sometimes finds what one is not looking for."
—Sir Alexander Fleming, Scottish biologist
and discoverer of penicillin in 1928

One chief complaint in the reviews of my first book, *Alzheimer's Disease: What If There Was a Cure? The Story of Ketones,* from researchers and physicians, including those from the Alzheimer's Association, is that the idea of using ketones as an alternative fuel to treat Alzheimer's disease hasn't had large clinical trials to back it up. While I agree that such studies are needed, how will they ever take place without awareness of the idea in the first place? Bringing awareness of ketones as an alternative fuel for the brain as a potential treatment for Alzheimer's and other neurodegenerative diseases was, and still is, my primary objective in writing these books.

Nearly seven years after I began trying to get this message out in June 2008, funding is still needed for the mass production and clinical testing of the ketone ester (a concentrated form of ketones) developed by Dr. Richard Veech, a senior scientist at the National Institutes of Health. The first clinical trial of a coconut oil and medium-chain triglyceride (MCT) oil combination for Alzheimer's disease is finally underway. My earliest messages, beginning just two weeks after Steve began to show dramatic improvement, were to scientists and politicians, asking them to look closely at the scientific rationale for providing ketones to the insulin-resistant brain and to study this urgently. (In Alzheimer's, insulin resistance prevents the brain cells from accepting glucose, their primary fuel.) It is as if the expectation, by even physicians who should know better, is that somehow such large-scale studies will magically materialize overnight or that someone would have thought of it a long time ago if there was any merit to it. They expect their patients, who will likely die or seriously worsen while waiting, to hold off on trying this dietary intervention until the results of clinical trials are in, even though the scientific basis justifies an individual trial on a "What-do-you-have-to-lose?" basis. Since coconut oil is a food, a staple in the diets of millions in other parts of the world, why can't a person serve as their own "control" (comparison subject) in a situation where the only other currently available alternative is continued worsening and death?

If the medical establishment had summarily dismissed important discoveries in the early part of the last century due to the expectation of having large, randomized, double-blind clinical trials before treatments were approved for general use, people might still be dying on a large-scale basis from bacterial infections. Likewise would type 1 and many type 2 diabetics have died from lack of insulin to control their blood sugar (glucose). The randomized double-blind clinical trial, now considered the "gold standard," was not recognized as such until the latter part of the twentieth century. These trials are used to help determine if a drug or medical device produces the desired effect in a real-world situation and whether there are adverse effects. No doubt they play a critical role in determining which drugs might be suitable for use to treat disease, however, they are not infallible.

Most drugs are not naturally occurring substances but are synthesized in a lab. Drugs reach not only the target organ but also most, if not all, other organs in the body, and may have toxic unintended consequences as a result. Nearly every drug on the market today carries a list of potential adverse effects that we need to be wary of, and even a higher risk of mortality with many of them. In spite of large, randomized, double-blind clinical trials of several thousand people, serious adverse effects sometimes become more evident after the drug is released and used by millions.

Rofecoxib (Vioxx), used primarily to treat arthritis, is just one example of a drug that was removed under pressure from the Food and Drug Administration (FDA) after just five years on the market. An estimated 20 million people used this drug and an unexpectedly high number of people had heart attacks while taking it before it was discontinued. It may even have been a trigger for the onset of Alzheimer's disease as was discovered in a study of people with mild cognitive impairment who were given Vioxx versus a placebo to try to prevent progression Alzheimer's disease. The people taking Vioxx had 1.46 times the risk of progressing to Alzheimer's than the people taking the placebo. This was acknowledged in a 2008 article in *Current Alzheimer's Research* in which the authors suggested various possibilities for why this progression occurred but could not confirm a mechanism with certainty. In an addendum to this article, the authors mention that similar studies with naproxen (Aleve) and celecoxib (Celebrex) were discontinued early due to cardiovascular safety concerns and a trend found in the analysis of early results for increased incidence of Alzheimer's disease in people randomized to take either of these drugs instead of the placebo (Aisen, 2008). Doctors prescribed Vioxx because it had purportedly passed the gold-standard test of the large, randomized, double-blind clinical trial.

Should dietary interventions have to follow this same not-necessarily gold standard before people try them and doctors suggest them, particularly when there is no better treatment to offer? What if the medical establishment was so mired down by such expectations when certain treatments, now widespread and taken for granted, were first put forth early in the last century?

Bear with me for a few minutes as I set the stage to make a critical point.

Penicillin, the first antibiotic, is just one example of a medication that did not meet the gold standard of the randomized double-blind clinical trial before it was accepted to treat infection, and the history is quite fascinating. In 1897, the young French physician Ernest Duchesne learned from Arab stable boys that they kept the saddles in a dark part of the stable to promote mold growth because it seemed to aid in the healing of saddle sores on the horses. He experimented with this and noted that the mold *Penicillium glaucium* eliminated the bacteria *Escherichia coli* in a culture. He further found that when he injected several piglets with a lethal dose of typhoid and this mold at the same time, they survived the infection. Unfortunately, his dissertation on these experiments was not accepted since he was only twenty-three; he entered the army and further progress on this idea died with Duchesne who became ill and expired from tuberculosis.

It was not for another thirty-one years until 1928, after a chance discovery, that Scottish biologist Sir Alexander Fleming resurrected the idea when he noted that the staphylococcus bacteria on a petri dish died when it was accidently contaminated with the mold *Penicillium notatum*. As fate would have it, this petri dish had actually been discarded with other dishes into a pail of disinfectant, but somehow missed entering the liquid. As Fleming removed it from the stack in the pail, he noticed an unusual pattern on the dish, found the mold contaminant, and his curiosity led him to further investigation. He soon learned that the mold juice would develop a bacteria-free ring around it when the petri dish was cultured with bacteria, even when the mold was diluted 800-fold. While others before Fleming had made similar observations, they didn't act on them. Fleming was the first to consider and then further explore the potential ramifications of this discovery. He called this substance "penicillin" and tried unsuccessfully for twelve years to find a chemist skilled enough to mass-produce it. He didn't, however, pursue the idea of using it to treat human infection directly, but instead focused his efforts with this mold to develop vaccines against common maladies such as whooping cough and influenza, since it would inhibit bacterial growth in cultures and allow these other organisms to multiply more readily.

In 1930, Cecil George Paine, a pathologist from Sheffield, England, did consider that human infections could respond to penicillin, and he successfully treated one adult and three babies who had serious eye infections caused by gonococcus, the bacteria that causes gonorrhea. After this, the great challenge was to mass-produce penicillin so that it could be used to treat the extraordinary number of people who needed it. At that point in time, it was difficult to make even enough to treat one serious infection in a human.

It was not until 1940 that this concept began to make any headway. Scientists Ernst Chain and Howard Florey in Oxford, England, were finally able to garner adequate funding to make enough purified penicillin to successfully treat streptococcus infection in mice, and repeat the experiment to verify this success. But, they needed considerably more to treat a person than a mouse and, still lacking adequate funding, through the efforts of a dozen lab personnel, they grew the penicillin mold in hundreds of flasks and bedpans and used dairy equipment to purify it, all for the purpose of treating a single human being. In 1941, they treated their first patient, Albert Alexander, a constable, who was scratched by a rose bush and developed a facial infection so severe that one eye had to be removed to relieve some of the pain. His infection began to improve just one day after beginning his treatment with penicillin; however, Florey and his group still did not have enough penicillin to take him to a full recovery, and, sadly, Albert relapsed and died.

It was the problem of securing adequate financing for mass production that held up the use of penicillin for widespread use for several more years. Ultimately, George Merck, a pharmaceutical maker in the United States, became interested in taking on the task. There were no large-scale randomized double-blind studies of penicillin before it became widely used. In fact, in March 1942, a single patient with streptococcus septicemia responded to treatment with penicillin, and in June 1942, another ten patients were successfully treated, launching a large-scale effort by the U.S. government a year later to begin mass production in anticipation of the need for prevention and treatment of infection in troops involved in the World War II efforts.

Just imagine how many hundreds of thousands, if not millions, of people died of an infection that could have been treated with penicillin between 1897 when the young scientist's idea was rejected and nearly a half century later in 1943 when it finally became widely available.

Similarly, it was twenty-one years from the time European researchers Oskar Minkowski and Josef von Mering discovered that removal of the pancreas caused type 1 diabetes in dogs in 1889, until it was suggested in 1910 that a single substance, now called insulin, was lacking, and yet another twelve more years until insulin was extracted from the pancreas, purified, and given for the first time to a single patient, a teenager, who improved dramatically. This was in 1922 and news spread like wildfire worldwide thereafter, based on this single case. Doctors did not wait for large-scale clinical trials to take place before prescribing insulin to their diabetic patients. Before insulin was available, even diabetics on a very strict high-fat, low-carb diet would live at most for one year. How many more would have died if doctors had decided to wait for results of large-scale randomized double-blind studies to prescribe insulin for their patients? For the individual person with diabetes, insulin would either work or not work. Why would control patients receiving the placebo have to die needlessly to prove that insulin works when it was already a given that everyone with type 1 diabetes will die without it? It is a given now that people with

Alzheimer's disease will inevitably deteriorate and die, so why can't a person suffering from this disease be offered an innocuous dietary intervention that might improve their condition, allowing them to effectively serve as their own control in the process?

I have digressed here to make a point. Over the course of modern medicine, it has been a common occurrence that a treatment presents itself by chance and that such treatment begins with improvement in a single patient. The proponents of these treatments are often met with obstacles, beginning with skepticism, and even outright ridicule on the part of many of their scientist peers, as well as a lack of support, both moral and financial, to bring the treatment into general use. Ultimately, it takes someone in authority who has the intellectual and financial expertise to make it happen, to recognize the potential of the treatment, and to bring it to fruition.

In 2000, Dr. Veech of the NIH, while developing a form of ketones that can be taken orally and that produces high levels, published the first research article suggesting that ketones could provide alternative fuel for the brain and improvement in people with Alzheimer's, Parkinson's, amyotrophic lateral sclerosis, multiple sclerosis, traumatic brain injury, and a plethora of other diseases that have in common the problem of decreased glucose uptake into brain and nerve cells. Fifteen years later, in spite of his own best efforts and the effort of others, he still lacks funding from his own governmental institution to produce more than the small amount he can make in his lab, much less to begin large scale testing in people with neurodegenerative diseases and traumatic brain injury. I cannot help but compare his struggle with getting recognition of the potential for ketones to treat millions of people to the very similar plight of Dr. Florey and his cohorts, who were relegated to making penicillin in bedpans in their lab to treat a single patient. They knew what they had but couldn't convince the powers-that-be for several years. How many hundreds of thousands of people died from a potentially easily treatable infection in the meantime?

In 2000, just after Dr. Veech's paper was published on the neuroprotective effect of ketones, geneticist Samuel Henderson, who lost his mother to Alzheimer's, had the idea that the ketones produced by consuming medium-chain triglycerides could provide alternative fuel to the brain and perhaps bring about improvement in people with Alzheimer's and mild cognitive impairment, which can lead to Alzheimer's. Dr. Henderson cofounded a small bio-tech company called Accera and embarked on a path to develop a patented medical food that had MCT oil as its active ingredient for people with Alzheimer's disease.

Recognition by the FDA as a medical food requires clinical trials and, in 2004, the report from their pilot study was published in which they documented cognitive improvement in Alzheimer's patients taking MCT oil (called AC-1202 in the study). This news did not receive attention from the media, physicians, or the public, and five more years passed before their product (now called Axona) was recognized in 2009 by the FDA as a medical food for this use. The active ingredient in Axona had already been on the shelf as coconut oil and MCT oil for decades and already carried GRAS (generally recognized as safe) status from the FDA; however, recognition as a medical food entitles Axona to be marketed for use in Alzheimer's disease.

Now, in 2015, eleven years after that first report, larger-scale studies of MCT oil are finally underway, as is the first study of a coconut oil and MCT oil combination in Alzheimer's patients. Many physicians have taken the approach that they want to wait the several years it will take for the results to come in to acknowledge the idea and support their patients who want to try this dietary intervention. Fortunately, for others suffering from these fatal diseases, their doctors have taken the path of reviewing the science, recognizing that it is feasible, and helping their patients by supporting and even suggesting that they try this approach. After all, what do they have to lose?

Introduction

*"A discovery is said to be an accident
meeting a prepared mind."*
—ALBERT SZENT-GYÖRGYI, HUNGARIAN SCIENTIST
AND DISCOVERER OF VITAMIN C, CIRCA 1931

There is an epidemic of Alzheimer's disease, less common dementias, and other neurodegenerative conditions, such as Parkinson's disease, multiple sclerosis, autism, and amyotrophic lateral sclerosis (ALS), that is growing exponentially. These days, nearly everyone has a family member or a friend with a family member struggling with Alzheimer's disease.

My husband, Steve, has early-onset Alzheimer's disease. He was an accountant and worked from home for my medical practice so that he could be there for our children when I had newborn emergencies to tend to. He was capable of creating the most detailed forms without errors, spent endless hours on the computer for work and for fun, read novel after novel, and was physically very active, whether kayaking for several miles at a time or working out in the yard. But at age fifty-one in 2001, he began to make payroll errors, missed tax report deadlines, and then could not remember if he had been to the bank or post office on a given day.

By 2003, he could no longer read a map and spent hours on end searching for "something" in the garage. He had to have one of the earliest computers when they first appeared and needed to upgrade as soon as the latest and fastest computer became available. In spite of spending hours on a computer every day for more than twenty-five years, by 2006, he could no longer remember how to use a mouse or even how to turn on a computer. He could no longer do any accounting, use a calculator, or even perform simple math, and had to give up driving that year after making a wrong turn and winding up three hours away on the other coast of Florida. He was more likely to take his lawn tractor apart than cut the grass with it. By the spring of 2008, he was on a downward spiral. He now had physical symptoms, such as tremors when he tried to talk or eat, a slow weird gait, and was unable to run. He had stopped reading, his favorite pastime, as the result of a visual disturbance that he later described as words "going into little boxes" and darting around on the page.

But then, in May 2008, something happened that altered the course of his disease for the better. It was completely by chance that I found it, but recognized it when I saw it because of what I do for a living. I am a neonatologist, a physician who cares for sick and premature newborns, and have practiced in newborn intensive care units in Florida for thirty years. While researching two clinical trial drugs, I happened upon a press release about a promising medical food working toward FDA approval that would not be available for another year. The makers claimed that this medical food, called Axona, improved memory and cognition in nearly half the people with Alzheimer's who were tested. The active ingredient in this food is a medium-chain triglyceride (MCT) oil known as caprylic triglyceride—a type of oil which, when consumed, is partly converted in the liver to ketones, an alternative fuel for brain cells. This is relevant because Alzheimer's is a type of diabetes of the brain. Areas of the brain affected by Alzheimer's develop insulin deficiency and insulin resistance, spreading eventually throughout the brain as the disease advances. Insufficient glucose uptake into brain and nerve cells also occurs in certain other types of dementia, Parkinson's disease, Huntington's disease, multiple sclerosis, autism, and many other conditions.

Glucose (also called blood sugar) is the primary fuel for the brain and insulin is required for glucose to be transported into the cells (Uemura, 2006). Insulin is also required at the junctions between brain cells (synapses) for the cells to maintain their connections and communicate with each other (Chiu, 2008). As insulin resistance develops, cells begin to malfunction and eventually die due to inadequate glucose entering the cells and the cells begin to lose their connections with each other. But the brain can use ketones as fuel when glucose is not readily available.

During starvation and with strict ketogenic diets, fat is metabolized to ketones, which are easily taken up by the cells of the brain and other organs and burned as fuel. In the course of my Internet research, I learned that MCT oil is extracted from coconut oil, the richest source of medium-chain triglycerides. I recognized MCT oil because we used it in the feedings of our very premature newborns to help them gain weight in the late 1970s and early 1980s. Since then, MCT oil and coconut oil have subsequently been added to virtually all infant formulas to mimic the fat content in breast milk. If I was not a neonatologist or pediatrician, I doubt that I would have been familiar with MCT oil and put two and two together, nor would I have known that it was readily available and that there was no need to wait for a prescription medical food to come on the market.

When Steve began to take just over two tablespoons of coconut oil, calculated to give an amount of medium-chain triglycerides equivalent to the tested dose in the medical food, he had a very dramatic response. Steve happened to be screening on successive days for two different clinical trials and his scores on a 30-point memory test (the Mini-Mental Status Exam) improved from 14 the day before to 18 just a few hours after taking coconut oil for the first time. His clock drawing improved very significantly at fourteen and thirty-seven days after starting coconut oil compared to the day before he began taking it (see Figure 1). Over the first few days, as we continued the coconut oil for breakfast and also began cooking with it later in the day, he had obvious improvements, such as increased alertness and less confusion in the morning, a return of his personality and sense of humor, more animation in his face, and the virtual disappearance of the tremors in his jaw and hands.

Over the next weeks to months, Steve's ability to complete his thoughts and participate in conversation gradually improved; his gait normalized and he was able to pick up his feet and run again;

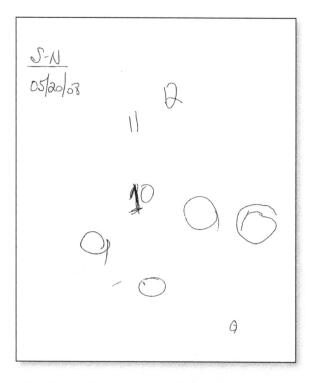

FIGURE 1. Three clocks drawn by Steve Newport one day before (above) and at fourteen (right, top) and thirty-seven days (right, bottom) after beginning a dietary intervention with coconut oil.

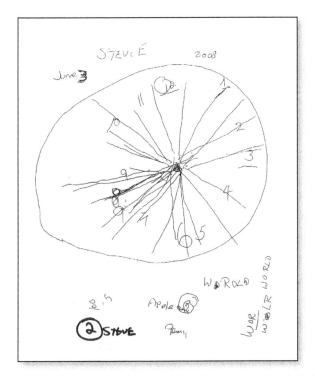

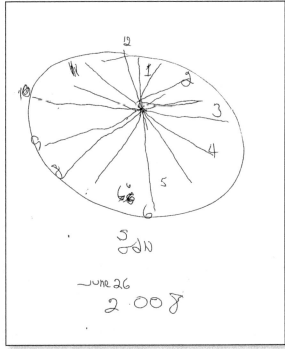

the visual disturbance that he was now able to describe went away and he was able to read again. He qualified for a clinical trial that he began about two months after starting the coconut oil. We later learned that he was in the placebo arm of the trial (those taking the inert substance) for at least the first twelve to fourteen months before crossing over to taking the drug. During the first year, his score on the cognitive section of the Alzheimer's Disease Assessment Scale improved by 6 points on a 75-point scale. And he improved by 14 points on the 78-point Activities of Daily Living test, reflected in an obvious improvement in his ability to care for himself and carry out tasks he was unable to do for quite some time, such as cutting the lawn and vacuuming.

By the end of the first year, his short-term memory had improved so much that he could tell me details of stories he had read several hours earlier. During the second year after starting coconut oil, he stabilized. The story of Steve's decline into Alzheimer's, his subsequent improvement while taking coconut and MCT oils, and setbacks along the way are detailed at length in my previous book, *Alzheimer's Disease: What If There Was a Cure? The Story of Ketones.*

By the time this book is published, it will be nearly seven years since Steve started taking coconut oil. About one-third of people with Alzheimer's eventually begin to have seizures, and unfortunately, Steve is one of them, beginning five years after starting coconut oil. Even though he may ultimately lose his battle with Alzheimer's, the course of his disease took an abrupt turn from a downward spiral to a climb out of the abyss. Steve went back in time at least two to three years in his disease process with improved quality of life for himself, for me as his wife and caregiver, and for our family. Who wouldn't want that no matter what disease we are dealing with and for however long it lasts?

Since starting to get the message out, I have received letters and e-mails from more than 400 people, mostly caregivers, reporting improvement in their loved ones with Alzheimer's disease, other dementias, Parkinson's disease, ALS, and other conditions. For some, these improvements were immediate and dramatic, and for others more gradual. Some people who were diagnosed with early-stage Alzheimer's, several people with Parkinson's, and a man with ALS have reported improvement followed by stabilization for three to four years. The key to this achievement is consistency: consuming coconut oil or MCT oil or both every day and probably several times a day. For all of these reasons, I continue to believe that until ketone esters (a concentrated form of ketones) and other ketone-containing drinks or foods are available, this dietary approach is well worth adopting both for people suffering from these conditions and as prevention for those who are at risk. At a recent international conference, one speaker stated that, since Alzheimer's disease mostly affects the elderly, if a treatment could be found that would delay the onset of Alzheimer's disease by five years, half the cases of this dreaded condition worldwide could be eliminated. Perhaps this is one of those hoped-for treatments.

When Steve improved in May 2008 in response to coconut oil, and with the medical food Axona a year away from FDA approval, I felt compelled to get the message out to everyone dealing with Alzheimer's and other diseases that might respond to this dietary approach. I wrote to politicians, the media, and many high-profile people about the medical food, the science behind it, Steve's response as just one example of someone who had a positive response, and the need to study this urgently. In July 2008, I wrote an article titled, "What If There Was a Cure for Alzheimer's Disease and No One Knew?" that has become circulated worldwide on the Internet and can be printed out for free from my website (www.coconutketones.com).

In the fall of 2011, *Alzheimer's Disease: What If There Was a Cure? The Story of Ketones* was published by Basic Health Publications. The primary intent of writing this book was to bring about

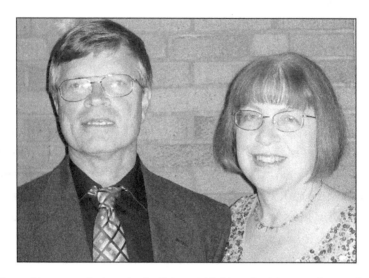

Steve Newport during the holidays with his wife, Mary, in December 2008, six months after starting coconut oil and MCT oil. By this time Steve's depression had lifted. He could now recognize and enjoy conversation with family, his tremors and stiff gait were gone, his memory was much improved, and he could read and enjoy gardening and other favorite activities once again.

awareness of the potential for treatment of Alzheimer's and other neurodegenerative diseases with dietary ketosis, through consumption of medium-chain triglycerides as coconut oil or MCT oil, or through ketone esters, which are on the path toward recognition by the FDA and can provide much higher levels of ketones. The main criticism of the book is that this approach needs clinical trials, and I wholeheartedly agree. Yet, how will clinical trials of coconut oil ever take place without awareness of the possibility in the first place?

Since the second edition of that book was published in 2013, results of a new retrospective study of patients taking Axona have been published, along with select case reports in a second article. These are discussed in more detail in Chapter 4. Two new animal studies of medium-chain triglycerides have also been published. The first study was from a group at the Byrd Alzheimer's Institute, in conjunction with the University of South Florida, in which two different transgenic mouse models were compared to non-transgenic mice, and in each group some mice received a ketogenic diet high in medium-chain triglycerides versus a control diet. The main finding of this study was a substantial and significant increase in motor performance, specifically in endurance, in all groups of mice on the ketogenic diet, along with persistent elevation of ketones and a lowering of blood glucose (Brownlow, 2013).

The second study, which was conducted at Memorial University of Newfoundland in Canada, found a significant effect by adding coconut oil to the mix when cultures of cortical rat neurons (nerve cells) were exposed to beta-amyloid peptide. (Beta-amyloid is a component of the plaques in Alzheimer's disease that is toxic to neurons.) The researchers found that about 30 percent more neurons survived in the cultures that contained higher amounts of coconut oil and concluded that "the presence of coconut oil can ameliorate the toxic effects of Abeta [beta-amyloid] on the neurons" (Nafar, 2014). While the results of a study in a petri dish must be taken with caution, since results might not translate to what occurs in a living brain, this is encouraging.

I am pleased to report that, in the summer of 2013, the Byrd Alzheimer's Institute launched a study of a mixture of coconut and MCT oils (Fuel for Thought from Cognate Nutritionals) versus a placebo in sixty-five people with mild to moderate Alzheimer's disease—the first study of its kind in people that I am aware of. This is a randomized double-blind clinical trial in which each participant will receive either Fuel for Thought or a placebo for three months and then cross over to the other for another three-month period; so, in effect, the participants will each serve as their own control. The study is expected to take two years or longer to complete. At least two larger studies of MCT oil in Alzheimer's disease are also in progress. In addition, the Alzheimer's Association is funding a three-year study at the University of Sherbrooke in Quebec of the effects of MCT oil on cognition and prevention of Alzheimer's in people with mild cognitive impairment. Clinical trials of ketone esters are imminent as well, with promising animal studies completed and others in progress, and at least one human pilot study planned in Oxford, England.

Ketogenic approaches are also undergoing intense study at the University of South Florida for treatment of cancer, ALS, wound healing, oxygen toxicity, epilepsy, and status epilepticus (continuous seizures). Results of these studies are now becoming available as fast as they can be completed and submitted to scientific journals (D'Agostino, 2013; Ari, 2014; Edwards, 2014; Poff, 2014; Seyfried, 2014). I believe strongly that ketones—whether obtained through coconut oil, MCT oil, ketone-containing drinks and foods, or special low-carb, high-fat ketogenic diets—can provide immediate and ongoing benefit as alternative fuel to the brain of infants, children, and adults who suffer from coma, traumatic brain injury, brain damage from lack of oxygen, severe hypoglycemic episodes, stroke, autism, and Down syndrome. I hope that animal and human clinical trials will be undertaken to study these as well.

While awaiting the results of these and other clinical trials, it is my goal that this message will reach the many millions dealing with this disease now, so that they become educated about the potential for ketones to provide alternative fuel for the brain and have the opportunity to decide for themselves, in conjunction with their physician, whether to undertake this approach. The use of coconut oil is too often dismissed out of hand by physicians who haven't actually studied the unusual and important properties of the medium-chain triglycerides found in coconut oil but instead conjure up old myths about coconut oil. I hope to counter these misconceptions so that physicians will help guide the use of this dietary intervention in their patients. The information is beginning to find its way to the mainstream of physicians. In December 2013, Medscape, an online educational resource for physicians, presented a continuing education program titled "Brain Glucose Hypometabolism, Ketosis, and Alzheimer's Disease: From Controversy to Consensus," which discusses the subject matter presented in this book.

One major deficit in the education of physicians in the United States is an overemphasis on treatment of diseases with drugs at the expense of education in nutrition. In medical school, I had a full semester of biochemistry, learning what happens to food metabolically after it is broken down and what happens to the molecules of fat, protein, and carbohydrates (sugar). But I had just a single afternoon of training in nutrition, and virtually no mention of specifically how eating the wrong foods can lead to diseases such as diabetes and how eating the right foods could potentially correct or prevent disease in the first place. The number of hours spent teaching new physicians the basics of nutrition has not increased much since I attended medical school in the 1970s, and the role of nutrition in treating their patients continues to be overlooked by very many physicians. There is a trend, however, toward alternative and integrative treatments and there are a growing number of physicians who consider nutrition as a vital component in treating their patients. Sadly, most of their education in this regard occurs independently of their medical school training.

The Coconut Oil & Low-Carb Solution for Alzheimer's, Parkinson's, and Other Diseases is designed as a companion to my previous book. *Alzheimer's Disease: What If There Was a Cure? The Story of Ketones* relays Steve's and my story, numerous caregiver reports, an intense discussion of the science of ketones and medium-chain triglycerides, as well some basics of how to incorporate coconut and MCT oils into the diet. This book gives an overview of the science yet focuses primarily on the practical aspects of undertaking this dietary intervention. The information is intended to serve as a quick reference for those who have read the previous book and will provide a basic understanding of the principles underlying this strategy to those who have not. In the interim years between these two books, there is growing recognition that Alzheimer's disease is a type of diabetes of the brain, which is very likely affected by excess carbohydrate intake. So, here, we will go beyond the use of coconut oil and look at choices for reducing carbohydrate intake and for eating a generally healthier diet to try to avoid diabetes altogether, or to lessen the effects for the person who already has this condition. This low-carb diet will not be an extreme diet but one that is realistic for the average person. With the focus on the practical, you will be able to begin these dietary interventions in short order.

A Dietary Plan to Overcome Insulin Resistance

A Quick-Start Guide to Using Coconut and Medium-Chain Triglyceride (MCT) Oils

No doubt most of you are anxious to begin, so here are some guidelines to help you or your loved one get started right away. More details and a question and answer section, as well as food ideas and recipes, are provided in later chapters in Part One. Even though coconut oil and MCT oil are foods, it is strongly recommended to get input from your physician before starting this dietary intervention, especially for people who suffer from chronic diseases that require medications. This dietary approach does not replace the other treatments prescribed by your physician and does not mean that you can now discontinue Alzheimer's medications without first discussing the issue with the physician. By now, many physicians who care for people with Alzheimer's disease and Parkinson's disease are aware of this dietary intervention and, hopefully, the rest will soon become educated on this subject. Many physicians have learned about this dietary plan for the first time from their patients.

WHO MAY BENEFIT AND HOW DOES IT HELP?

This dietary intervention may be appropriate for treatment and also for prevention of certain conditions. People most likely to benefit are those who have or are at risk for a neurodegenerative disease that involves decreased glucose uptake into neurons and other nerve cells, and also people who have prediabetes or already have type 1 or 2 diabetes and are at higher risk than average of developing dementia. Because insulin is needed to get glucose into most cells, the cells may malfunction and eventually die due to lack of fuel. When foods with medium-chain triglycerides are eaten, the liver converts part of the oil to ketones, which act as an alternative fuel to glucose for brain cells and other organs. Conditions that may respond to this approach include Alzheimer's disease (also known as diabetes of the brain) and some other less common dementias, Parkinson's disease, diabetes, ALS, multiple sclerosis, autism, Down syndrome, and Huntington's disease.

There are a number of uncommon conditions that also involve decreased glucose uptake in the brain or other organs that could respond (for a list of the conditions, see Appendix 1). Your physician should be able to help you discover if this dietary intervention is appropriate for you or your loved one.

Also, people who have bipolar disease, and memory issues or "brain fog," whether related to aging or not, might consider trying this approach. I have heard from many people describing themselves in this way who feel coconut oil has helped them feel better and think more clearly.

Some rare conditions involve a problem of fat metabolism in which the use of coconut oil or oil and MCT oil may not be appropriate and may even worsen the condition (see also Appendix 1 for a list of these conditions). Therefore, consultation with your physician is very important.

AN OVERVIEW:
DIETARY CHOICES TO RAISE KETONE LEVELS

The primary goal with this undertaking is to increase ketones in the circulation (called ketosis) so that they will reach brain cells to provide an alternative fuel to cells that are not using glucose effectively. The levels you are aiming for are very low compared to the levels that occur during diabetic ketoacidosis, a potentially life-threatening condition that is often confused with the term ketosis. It is extremely unlikely that these dietary interventions would cause someone to go into diabetic ketoacidosis, since the levels of ketones are at least ten to twenty times higher in that condition, which also only occurs in diabetics with out-of-control blood sugar due to the absence of insulin (most often new, unrecognized type 1 diabetics or in diabetics who are not taking their insulin).

There are a number of dietary measures that can be taken to raise ketone levels alone or in combination with each other. Which you choose will largely depend on the daily life situation of you or

SOME CAVEATS

- It is strongly recommended that you discuss beginning this intervention, or any other significant dietary change, with your physician first. This is particularly true for people who suffer from chronic diseases and/or are taking medications.

- Do not stop any medications without specific discussion with your physician.

- Do not use coconut oil if you are allergic to coconut.

- If you are on insulin or diabetes medication, be sure to monitor your blood sugar closely as some people will experience a drop in blood sugar, particularly when taking larger amounts of coconut or MCT oil. Discuss this dietary intervention with your doctor so that your medications can be adjusted if necessary.

- If you have severe liver disease or liver failure or certain rare enzyme defects involving fat metabolism, raising ketones by any of these dietary choices is not recommended for you.

your affected loved one. Here are the currently available choices with more details to follow shortly:

- Ketogenic and low-carb diets
- Coconut oil or palm kernel oil
- MCT oil
- Mixture of coconut and MCT oils (prepared at home)
- Commercially prepared, over-the-counter mixture of coconut and MCT oils
- Axona, an FDA-approved prescription medical food

Hopefully, in the not-too-distant future, we will have the option of commercially prepared ketone-containing drinks and foods that will raise ketone levels considerably higher than large amounts of coconut oil, MCT oil, or Axona. Studies working toward FDA approval are in progress (see preface for details).

Ketogenic and Low-Carb Diets

Reducing carbohydrates in the diet is an important key to prevention and could potentially slow down the progression of diseases of insulin resistance, such as Alzheimer's disease. Ketogenic diets are low in carbohydrates (particularly refined carbohydrates like sugar and processed foods) and high in fats, and can be used alone or in combination with other choices. While the other choices below will raise ketone levels independent of the amount of carbohydrates in the diet in most people, adopting a lower-carbohydrate diet can enhance the effectiveness of these other measures by raising ketone levels even more. A ketogenic diet may also be a viable option for the rare person who simply cannot tolerate even small amounts of coconut and MCT oils or for someone who does not respond to coconut or MCT oil, since the diet can generate higher levels than either coconut or MCT oil. The various forms of a ketogenic diet and specific guidelines for reducing carbohydrates in the diet will be discussed in Chapter 2.

KETOGENIC AND LOW-CARB DIET QUICK TIPS

- May prevent or slow down progression of Alzheimer's and other diseases involving insulin resistance.

- Provides an option for people unable to tolerate coconut and MCT oils.

- Can generate higher levels of ketones than either coconut or MCT oil.

- Enhances effectiveness of other ketone-producing measures by further raising ketone levels.

Coconut Oil or Palm Kernel Oil

Coconut oil is extracted from the kernel or meat of coconuts. It is the richest natural source of medium-chain triglycerides, containing nearly 60 percent of these ketone-producing fatty acids. Coconut oil is what started me on my discovery of what ketones can do for someone with Alzheimer's, resulting in at least two to three better quality years for my husband, Steve, and our family. The people I have heard from who have experienced long-term stabilization over two or more years have been taking coconut oil consistently every day, and usually several times a day. An important fact about coconut oil is that it is 50 percent lauric acid. Lauric acid is one of the medium-chain triglycerides and is known to be antimicrobial against certain viruses, bacteria, protozoa (single-celled organisms), and fungi (yeasts). With considerable evidence that particular microorganisms could trigger Alzheimer's disease, Steve and I decided to keep coconut oil as a staple in our diet rather than using only MCT oil, which is prepared to contain little or no lauric acid.

Palm kernel oil is extracted from the seed of the palm fruit. It is not readily available in the United States but may be in more tropical parts of the world. It contains about 54 percent of its fats as medium-chain triglycerides and so the guidelines hereafter for coconut oil would apply to palm kernel oil as well.

Coconut oil is readily available in most natural food stores, most Asian markets, and also now in many mainstream grocery stores. As far as producing ketones as fuel for the brain, it does not matter whether the oil is refined or not, organic or not; although partially hydrogenated coconut oil with harmful trans fats should be strictly avoided, since consuming them could undermine your efforts to improve brain health. An easy way to determine whether trans fats are in the oil is to look at the nutrition information label on the container. If trans fats are listed or the ingredients state that the oil is hydrogenated or partially hydrogenated, put it back on the shelf and look for another product. Organic unrefined, or virgin, coconut oil is less processed and may contain some nutrients not found in refined coconut oil, so some may prefer the organic oil for this reason. For those on a low fixed income, the choice of what type of coconut oil to use may be a matter of one's budget, and, for the few who do not care for the odor of coconut, the refined oil may be the way to go. Check the Resources section for a listing of websites offering coconut oil and coconut oil products.

Coconut oil is tasteless but often enhances the flavors of foods it is added to. It melts at 76° Fahrenheit (F) (25° Celsius) and, at this temperature and above, is a clear or slightly yellow liquid. At 75°F (24°C) and below, coconut oil is a white or yellowish semi-solid that can easily be spooned out of the container. As the coconut oil goes from liquid to solid, it may look like white clouds floating in clear liquid. There is no need to worry—the oil has not gone bad. The shelf life of coconut oil is at least two years at room temperature and it is so stable that it does not need to be refrigerated. In fact, if you decide to refrigerate it, you may need a chisel to get it out of the container! I learned this the hard way.

Heating does not alter the composition of coconut oil unless it begins to smoke. The best way to use coconut oil is to cook with it or to put it into or on a food that is warm. It will quickly melt down, or you can simply melt it before adding it to a food that is cool or at room temperature. Just be aware that the oil quickly hardens when added to cold foods. Coconut oil is unaffected by brief microwaving, so a few spoonfuls can be placed in a small bowl and put in the microwave on high for 10 to 15 seconds. As an alternative, the bowl of coconut oil can be placed into a container of hot water and left to stand until it melts. There is only a very slight difference between the volume of a level tablespoon of solid versus liquid coconut oil.

The one precaution about cooking with coconut oil is that it tends to smoke at greater than 350°F (175°C). That's quite low compared to many other oils. So, when cooking with it on the stove, keep the temperature at medium heat or less. If a higher

---

COCONUT OIL QUICK TIPS

- Store at room temperature.

- Becomes chunky in cold foods.

- Mix into something warm or pre-warm before mixing into cool foods.

- Use medium heat or lower when cooking on stovetop to avoid smoking; if higher heat is needed, add a small amount of olive, canola, or peanut oil.

- Bake in oven at a maximum temperature of 350°F or lower when basted on food to avoid smoking; if mixed into food, higher temperatures are fine.

temperature is needed, a small amount of olive oil, canola oil, or peanut oil can be added to the pan to keep the coconut oil from smoking. In the oven, coconut oil will be fine at higher temperatures if it is mixed into the food, but, if the oil is painted on to the food, stay at 350°F or below to avoid smoking.

Some people experience intestinal upset (indigestion or sudden explosive diarrhea) if they try to consume too much coconut oil when starting, so a good approach is to begin by adding one-half to one level teaspoon (about 2.5 to 5 milliliters [ml] or grams) to food two or three times a day. If this is tolerated without a problem, then increase by this same amount every two to three days as tolerated. If there is some diarrhea, I suggest backing off to the previous level, waiting for several days, and then increasing the amount even more gradually. The more coconut oil one consumes, the more ketones will be produced; ultimately, the total daily amount to strive for will be determined by how much the individual can tolerate. For most people, this will likely be about three to six level tablespoons of coconut oil per day, although I know of many who are taking more, as much as nine to twelve tablespoons per day divided into three to four servings. Chapter 3 supplies information about coconut milk, grated coconut, and other coconut products that can be used in place of coconut oil.

Another suggestion is to substitute coconut oil for other fats in the diet and also to reducing the amount of carbohydrate in the diet. If you simply add the oil to the diet, the added calories could result in weight gain, although for some people this may be desirable. Another reason to cut out or reduce portions of carbohydrates is to keep blood sugar from spiking repeatedly, thereby keeping insulin levels lower in an effort to stop, or at least slow down, further development of the problem of insulin resistance. High levels of insulin could interfere with production of ketones, which is another good reason to control carbohydrate intake. Specific suggestions for reducing carbohydrate intake will appear in Chapter 2 on diet.

MCT Oil

Medium-chain triglyceride oil is commonly abbreviated as MCT oil. The oil is typically extracted from coconut oil or palm kernel oil and has a shelf life of two years or longer if kept in a closed container at 74°F (23°C) or below. It has been used in infant formulas for decades and can be found in many natural food stores, particularly those that cater to bodybuilders, who use it to increase lean muscle mass. Unlike most other fats, MCT oil does not require bile salts to be digested. Because of this, it might be tolerated better than coconut oil by some people who have had their gallbladder removed or who have malabsorption problems, such as ulcerative colitis or Crohn's disease. A number of studies show that MCT oil may be useful for losing weight and it is often used for this reason as well. MCT oil is not stored as fat and, when consumed, part of it is converted to ketones and the rest is used immediately as fuel by other organs of the body, including the brain, muscles, and heart. The fatty acids in MCT oil might also provide alternative fuel for the brain (discussed in Chapter 4).

MCT oil can be purchased online from a number of different websites (see the Resources section) for very reasonable prices, from $17 to $70 per quart. Most MCT oils are a mixture of four medium-chain triglycerides and usually at least 60 percent caprylic triglyceride, the active ingredient in the prescription medical food Axona (discussed shortly), which is believed to be the most ketogenic of the medium-chain triglycerides. The MCT oil in Fuel for Thought (also discussed shortly) is caprylic triglyceride, and there is nearly 100 percent caprylic triglyceride in CapTri MCT Oil (from www.parillo.com); both are over-the-counter products. Caprylic triglyceride, however, is also the most likely to cause diarrhea, so some may tolerate the MCT oil mixture better.

MCT oil is clear, colorless, and tasteless, and is liquid at room temperature, although it will tend to solidify in the refrigerator. It is possible to cook with MCT oil on the stove; however, its smoke point is 320°F (160°C) and it tends to foam, so a low to medium heat is the limit. It can be mixed into foods that are baked in the oven but will smoke if painted on to the food above 320°F. MCT oil does not harden as readily as coconut oil when added to cool foods, which makes it especially amenable to using in smoothies and on a salad alone or in conjunction with another salad oil and balsamic vinegar or lemon. MCT oil can be mixed into many other foods, warm or cold.

A Japanese company, Nisshin Oillio, has developed a product, which has been on the market there since 2004, called Healthy Resetta Oil (www.nisshin-oillio.com/english/products/index.shtml). It contains MCT oil that is slightly changed by the addition of a long-chain fatty acid, which allows it to be used for cooking at higher temperatures and also without foaming. This special oil is combined with canola oil in the final product. Healthy Resetta Oil is one of only 100 foods that carry a healthy food label from the Japanese government; a designation it receives because medium-chain triglycerides are not stored as fat and can therefore be used to avoid weight gain. This company has been studying and producing MCT oil for over twenty years. The oil is also now available in the United States. They are also creating other tasty MCT foods.

From the reports I have received, more people experience intes-

---

MCT OIL QUICK TIPS

- Stays liquid when stored at room temperature.
- Mixes easily with most cold foods without solidifying.
- Cook on stove top over low-medium heat to avoid smoking.
- Bake in oven at a maximum temperature of 320°F or lower.

tinal upset, particularly sudden explosive diarrhea, with MCT oil than with coconut oil when new to taking it. For this reason it is a good idea, as with coconut oil, to begin by adding one-half to one teaspoon (2.5 to 5 ml or grams) to food two or three times a day. If the oil is tolerated without a problem, then increase by this same amount every two to three days as tolerated. If there is some diarrhea, once again, I suggest backing off to the previous level, waiting for several days, and then increasing even more gradually, perhaps every week or two. The total daily amount to strive for will depend on how much the individual can tolerate. Since MCT oil is more concentrated than coconut oil and is more likely to cause diarrhea, the limit will likely be somewhere around three to four tablespoons per day divided into three to four servings. The key to tolerating MCT oil is to take it with food. If it is incorporated into a serving of food or drink that will take twenty minutes or so to eat, all the better, since it will be digested more slowly this way.

Table 1.1 summarizes the guidelines for starting coconut oil and MCT oil.

TABLE 1.1. QUICK-START GUIDELINES FOR COCONUT OIL AND MCT OIL		
	AMOUNT	**HOW OFTEN**
Begin with	$^1/_2$–1 level teaspoon (2.5–5 ml or grams) per serving	2 to 3 times a day with food
If tolerated, increase by	$^1/_2$–1 level teaspoon (2.5–5 ml or grams) per serving	Every 2 to 3 days
Increase to	Coconut oil: 1–2 tablespoons (15–30 ml or grams) per serving, or more, as tolerated	3 to 4 times a day with food
	MCT oil: 4 teaspoons (20 ml or grams) per serving	3 to 4 times a day with food

Home-Prepared Mixture of Coconut and MCT Oils

Two months after Steve started consuming coconut oil and received the results of his ketone levels, we began experimenting with mixing MCT oil and coconut oil. After taking just coconut oil in the morning, Steve's ketone levels peaked at three hours and were nearly gone after eight to nine hours right before dinnertime, while his ketone levels with just MCT oil were higher but gone within three hours. It seemed reasonable then that a mixture of MCT oil and coconut oil would result in higher levels and longer-lasting levels, so that some ketones should always be circulating and available to the brain if this mixture is taken three to four times a day. After some experimentation, we settled on a mixture of four parts MCT oil to three parts coconut oil. The recipe for this mixture appears in Chapter 5, but I suggest that you begin by taking *either* coconut oil or MCT oil, rather than mixing them together. This way you will have a better idea of which oil is causing the problem, should you not tolerate it. After trying coconut or MCT oil first, if you choose to use the MCT and Coconut Oil 4:3 Mixture, it can be substituted for MCT oil in any of the recipes in Chapter 5. The mixture stays liquid at room temperature and does not tend to clump like coconut oil when added to cold foods.

MCT/COCONUT MIXTURE QUICK TIPS

- Remains liquid at temperature.
- Does not clump like coconut oil when added to cold foods.
- May provide higher and longer-lasting levels of ketones.
- Use only after first trying coconut oil and MCT oil.

Commercially Prepared, Over-the-Counter Mixture of Coconut and MCT Oils

If the affected loved one is in assisted living or if you are looking for convenience, eat out a lot, travel, or are otherwise not likely to use coconut oil for cooking or in foods, an ultra-convenient alternative is to try a product such as Fuel for Thought from Cognate Nutritionals (www.fuelforthought.co). The formulation is a creamy fruit-flavored mixture of coconut oil, highly enriched with MCT oil. It is packaged in two-serving bottles that can be taken as is or added to other foods or liquids. Fuel for Thought contains no preservatives or other additives but can be kept at room temperature on the day it is opened. Each serving has more than double the ketone-producing medium-chain triglycerides as three tablespoons of coconut oil. For those in assisted living, the doctor may be willing to write an order for the staff to administer the product at mealtimes. As with coconut oil and MCT oil, start with a small amount of the mixture, such as one-quarter (or even less) of the serving bottle to see how well it is tolerated, and then increase slowly. This over-the-counter product is being used in the ongoing coconut oil–MCT oil study in Alzheimer's at the Byrd Alzheimer's Institute at the University of South Florida (noted earlier). It is currently available in the United States but should be obtainable in other parts of the world soon.

Another product, developed by Alpha Health Products (www.alphahealth.ca) in Canada, called MCT Coconut Gourmet Salad Oil, combines MCT oil with virgin coconut oil in the four-to-three ratio that Steve and I have used. An unrefined omega-3-rich vegetable oil is also added and gives a pleasant nutty taste. This oil mixture is liquid and stable at room temperature due to its high-MCT content and will easily combine with lemon or vinegar to make salad dressing.

COMMERCIALLY PREPARED MCT/ COCONUT MIXTURE QUICK TIPS

- Convenient alternative that requires no cooking or preparation.
- Is liquid and stable at room temperature.
- Easily added to foods or liquids.

Axona: Prescription Medical Food

Even though the use of coconut and MCT oils are dietary in nature, many people and their physicians are more accepting of treatments that have undergone clinical trials and have received Food and Drug Administration (FDA) recognition. If this is the case, Axona (www.about-axona.com) is an option to consider since it can be prescribed and monitored by one's personal physician. If it were not for the development of this product and a press release about it in 2008, it is unlikely that I would have learned about the potential for coconut oil to produce ketones and help people diagnosed with Alzheimer's and other diseases. The active ingredient in Axona is caprylic triglyceride, a medium-chain fatty acid that is usually extracted from coconut or palm kernel oil. At present, a once-a-day

---

AXONA QUICK TIPS

- Available by prescription only.
- Powdered form of medium-chain triglycerides.
- FDA approved for once-a-day dose.
- Can be supplemented with coconut and MCT oils at meals.

dose is recommended because that is the dosing regimen that was studied. Two or three doses a day could potentially provide more benefit and further studies could answer that question soon. Many people supplement their morning dose of Axona with either coconut oil or MCT oil or both at other meals.

HELPFUL STARTERS

Here are some easy suggestions to help you get started on the journey toward incorporating coconut and MCT oils into the diet.

Keep a Journal

To help you decide if using medium-chain triglycerides is effective, it can be helpful to keep a journal. Shortly after it became obvious that Steve was improving, my sister Angela suggested that I start a journal, and this has been invaluable. About two weeks after Steve's first dose of coconut oil, as he improved, it occurred to me that I might forget what he was like before he started taking it. I wrote several pages describing my observations about his symptoms, not only related to memory and cognition but also effects on each of his senses, physical symptoms, our interactions with each other, and some of the rather odd things he would do. In the beginning, I made notes every day about how much oil he was taking, how we were using it in foods and recipes, and of course, how he was doing.

At this point, nearly seven years later, I make journal entries every so often, noting any significant changes to Steve's medications and diet, and in his functioning, whether positive or negative.

For people trying this dietary intervention, a journal could be useful for gauging how a loved one is responding over a period of time. At the very least I suggest that you record the following:

- Dates of your entries in the journal.

- Observations (general and specific) about the person's symptoms prior to adding medium-chain triglycerides to the diet.

- Starting dose, including how much and how often.

- Each increase in dose, including how much and how often.

- Any side effects, such as diarrhea or indigestion, and anything unusual for that person.

- Methods of use (straight from the spoon, mixed into foods, cooking with the oil, etc.) and what foods you are using with it.

- Observations (general and specific) about changes in the individual for better or worse.

- If the person is diabetic, record blood sugar measurements as well to see if there is a noticeable trend. This information could be useful to help the doctor monitor and possibly adjust or eliminate insulin and/or diabetes medications.

At any point in time, you can look back at your journal entries and have a better idea of whether your loved one has improved, seems to be about the same, or has gotten worse. With or without formal testing, these entries will help you decide whether this intervention is helpful.

Quick and Easy Food Ideas

When people first learn about coconut oil for Alzheimer's and other neurodegenerative diseases, many assume that it must be taken right off the spoon as if it is a medication. Sure, you can take it that way if it is the most convenient way for you and you don't have an overactive gag reflex! Steve has taken his mixture of coconut and MCT oils straight many times this way and it doesn't bother him to do this whatsoever. But there is no reason to have to take it this way.

Coconut oil is a food and, like most other oils, can be used to cook with on the stove or in the oven; it can easily be spread or poured over or mixed into many other foods too. As noted earlier, coconut oil works best with foods that are warmer than room temperature. MCT oil can also be used in combination with other foods. MCT oil is liquid at room temperature and tends to work better than coconut oil with cool or cold foods. MCT oil is particularly good for use in smoothies and as a salad dressing alone or with other ingredients, whereas coconut oil is not quite as easy to use this way. On the other hand, MCT oil is not particularly great in the skillet because it smokes and foams at a lower temperature than coconut oil. When coconut and MCT oils are combined, the mixture stays liquid at room temperature and behaves more like MCT oil than coconut oil in that it also works well with foods that are cool or cold, such as in smoothies.

Here are a few ideas for how to start working these medium-chain triglycerides into meals and snacks. Chapter 5 contains recipes for most of the suggestions here, in addition to many other dishes.

Breakfast Ideas

- Mix coconut oil or MCT oil or powder into coffee or tea; the oil will float to the top and many people find it easy to take it this way.

- Use coconut oil in the skillet to make scrambled eggs, an omelet, or a frittata; the oil will be absorbed into the eggs and other ingredients.

- Mix MCT oil into skim milk and drink it or pour it on hot or cold whole-grain cereals.

- Mix MCT oil or MCT and Coconut Oil 4:3 Mixture into coconut milk.

- Add MCT oil or MCT and Coconut Oil 4:3 Mixture, and/or coconut milk into smoothies.

- Add melted coconut oil, MCT oil, or MCT and Coconut Oil 4:3 Mixture into cottage cheese, ricotta, or yogurt.

- Mix grated coconut into cottage cheese, ricotta, or yogurt.

- Ideally it is best to avoid or at least minimize the intake of carbohydrate foods like breads and cereals to prevent a spike in insulin early in the morning; however, if your loved one is resistant to this idea, here are some other breakfast ideas:
  - Mix coconut or MCT oil into warm oatmeal or other hot whole-grain cereal. (Avoid packaged instant versions that have more sugar and additives and fewer nutrients.)
  - Use diluted coconut milk on whole-grain hot or cold cereals.
  - Add grated, unsweetened coconut to hot or cold whole-grain cereals.
  - Spread coconut oil or coconut butter on whole-grain toast, English muffins, and bagels; mix into grits or toss into pasta.

Lunch and Dinner Ideas

- Mix coconut oil or MCT oil or powder into coffee or tea.

- Mix MCT oil into skim milk and drink it.

- Use coconut oil in the skillet to make scrambled eggs, an omelet, or a frittata.

- Mix coconut oil or MCT oil into soups, stews, or chili.

- Use coconut oil in the skillet to sauté vegetables or to toss with already prepared warm vegetables.

- Use MCT oil or MCT and Coconut Oil 4:3 Mixture on salad. You can also mix these oils with other salad dressings or make your own salad dressings with them.

- Use coconut oil in the skillet to cook chicken or fish.

- Use coconut oil instead of other oils to brown ground beef, pork, or turkey.

- Paint coconut oil on salmon or other fish and bake (at 350°F or less).

- Paint coconut oil on vegetables and bake (at 350°F or less).

- Mix coconut oil, MCT oil, or MCT and Coconut Oil 4:3 Mixture into warm marinara, spaghetti sauce, or gravy.

- Toss coconut oil, MCT oil, or MCT and Coconut Oil 4:3 Mixture into warm gluten-free pasta or noodles.

- Add MCT oil or MCT and Coconut Oil 4:3 Mixture, and/or coconut milk into smoothies.

- Use coconut oil to replace part or all of butter or vegetable oils in nearly any recipe.

Snacks and Treats

- Have a handful of flaked coconut or coconut chips.

- Drink a glass of coconut milk.

- Mix a glass of skim milk with MCT oil or MCT and Coconut Oil 4:3 Mixture.

- Make a smoothie with MCT oil or MCT and Coconut Oil 4:3 Mixture, and/or coconut milk.

- Have some trail mix with flaked coconut, dried cherries and/or other dried fruit in small quantities.

- Make popcorn in coconut oil, or top it with coconut oil or a mixture of butter and coconut oil.

- Nibble on several pieces of coconut fudge or coconut-peanut butter fudge with nuts or grated coconut for variety.

- Have a scoop of coconut milk-based ice cream (any flavor).

- Add coconut milk and grated coconut to a dish of ricotta cheese and sweeten to taste with stevia (an herbal sweetener that does not have the same effect on the body as sugar), and top with nuts.

What Can You Expect?

If this dietary intervention is to make a difference, it is important to begin very slowly so that the person taking the oil is not immediately discouraged by a serious and embarrassing bout of diarrhea. It is also important to include the oil in the diet *every day* consistently. This process is much like a car, in that, if there is no gas in the tank, it won't run. I have heard from caregivers of a number of people who had a good response to coconut oil, and then discontinued its use for one reason or another (travel, a relative's "concern" about coconut oil, etc.) with an obvious, almost immediate decline within a day or so. The good news is that they report when the oil is restarted, the improvements generally return. Ketones are literally "fuel for the brain."

Go One Giant Step Further: A Low-Carb Diet

Are you old enough to remember that when we wanted to lose weight, we were advised to cut out sweets and starchy foods? Effectively, we were putting ourselves on a lower-carb diet. This was the "way to go" until the low-fat diet—a diet that by default is high in carbohydrates—became dogma in the latter part of the twentieth century. Before this dogma prevailed, extremely obese people were a rarity in the United States and much less common-place than today, where two-thirds of adults are considered over-weight or obese. Losing weight is a constant topic of conversation among most of my friends and coworkers. We are tempted by a never-ending barrage of sugary foods and drinks in the workplace, in television and magazine ads, and in the aisles and checkout stands of grocery stores.

Here we are going to switch gears and go back to a time not too long ago when people ate more fat and less sugar, when type 2 diabetes and Alzheimer's disease were much less common, and when twenty to forty pounds of extra weight was considered "a big problem" compared with 100 or even 200 pounds today. Most people who read this book will be caring for someone with Alzheimer's, or dealing with the disease personally, or worrying about developing the disease. If your loved one is elderly, it is unlikely that he or she will respond well to the idea of embarking on an extreme all-or-nothing type of diet that begins with a crash induction period like some of the recent fad diets that are intended for maximum weight loss. Instead, our goals will simply be to make healthier food choices as we transition to a sensible and realistic reduction in carbohydrates, while maintaining an adequate protein intake and incorporating coconut oil and other healthy fats into the diet.

You can make the transition to this diet for you or your loved ones as gradually as you wish. How far you take the carbohydrate reduction is completely up to you. You may or may not lose weight with this diet depending on how much food you choose to eat. If you deviate from the diet now and then with a high-carb treat, all is not lost. Simply remind yourself that if you can avoid an excessive intake of added sugars and eliminate refined carbohydrates as much as possible from your diet, along with other food additives, as a long-term strategy, you will greatly increase your odds of living healthier as well as keeping Alzheimer's and diabetes at bay.

CARBOHYDRATES, ALZHEIMER'S, AND DIABETES

It is important to think of your loved one with Alzheimer's or yourself if you are at risk as diabetic because, in a very real sense, this is true. The areas of the brain that are affected by Alzheimer's manifest insulin deficiency and insulin resistance, which result in decreased glucose uptake into the mitochondria (energy factories) of the cells, and eventually cell malfunction and death. In addition, a number of other conditions are associated with poor glucose uptake into areas of the brain that could represent insulin resistance as well; they just haven't been studied as extensively as Alzheimer's in that regard yet. Reducing carbohydrates in the diet is key to preventing and potentially slowing down the processes that result in insulin resistance, and ultimately in the symptoms of these dreaded diseases.

The Big Benefits of Going Low-Carb

Many of the carbohydrates we eat today come from added sugars, especially sucrose (also called table sugar), and high-fructose corn syrup. Less than 200 years ago, table sugar was available only to the wealthiest people and, as such, it has come very late in our evolutionary process. When we eat sugar, our insulin levels increase accordingly because insulin is needed to utilize glucose in cells as fuel or to store it as glycogen in the liver and muscles for later use. Simple carbohydrates, sometimes called simple sugars, found in refined sugar and most processed foods, increase glucose levels in the blood quickly and tend to cause insulin levels to spike; whereas complex carbohydrates, or complex sugars, found in whole grains, are digested more slowly and insulin rises more slowly accordingly. There are a multitude of potential benefits that come with keeping carbohydrate intake within reasonable limits and choosing foods that do not cause insulin levels to spike. Here are a few:

- Reducing carbohydrates can help break a carbohydrate addiction. After a few days on a low-carb diet, the constant feeling of hunger and craving for more carbohydrate-rich foods will begin to subside and eventually become a thing of the past. I can tell you from personal experience that going from being a carboholic to rarely craving sweets is a wonderful feeling.

- If you are not diabetic, reducing carbohydrates can help you avoid becoming diabetic.

- If you are already prediabetic or suffer from type 2 diabetes, reducing carbohydrates can help lower your insulin levels, reverse the trend toward insulin resistance, and avoid a multitude of complications that may occur over time, including mental decline, dementia, kidney failure, blindness, and/or amputations related to poor circulation.

- Reducing carbohydrates may lower the risk of cancer. Cancer cells thrive on sugar and depriving them of sugar could help shrink or kill a tumor and prevent the cells from spreading from one part or organ to another (metastases). Research in this important area is in progress. Maintaining a low-carb diet in general could potentially discourage cancerous tumors from forming in the first place.

- Reducing carbohydrates may diminish symptoms of diseases caused by inflammation. Chronically high sugar levels can result in inflammation, which is a common denominator in many neurodegenerative disorders, including Alzheimer's disease, Parkinson's disease, ALS, and autism. Inflammation in blood vessel walls is common in people who have high blood pressure and have had a heart attack or a stroke. Arthritis often involves inflammation of the joints, and less sugar overall could potentially reduce the pain that comes with this condition.

- Reducing sugar can help produce healthier, longer-living cells and tissues, and ultimately a longer life. When sugar binds to proteins, fats, and amino acids (a process called glycation), it alters their shape such that they are may not function normally. Proteins that have undergone glycation can link together and cause damage to surrounding tissues. A high-carbohydrate intake promotes excessive glycation and may speed up the process of aging and some of the common disease processes associated with aging. One obvious outward benefit would be less sagging and wrinkling of the skin as we age but our internal organs would benefit as well.

- Reducing sugar could lower serum triglyceride (blood fat) levels, since too much sugar may raise serum triglyceride levels well above normal and result in greater risk of heart disease. A common misconception is that high-serum triglyceride levels must be caused by eating a lot of fat, but, in reality, for most people, the main culprit is eating too much sugar and too many calories. Fructose, the sugar in fruit, does not convert to glucose after it is digested but rather is largely converted to triglycerides. Simple everyday table sugar is roughly half glucose and half fructose. High-fructose corn syrup, found in a multitude of soda, sugary drinks, and packaged foods, is proportionately even higher in fructose than table sugar (55 to 90 percent). If you drink Coca-Cola or Mountain Dew and you have a high-triglyceride level, consider giving the axe to these drinks. If the axe is too drastic, then wean off them one can at a time. Humans didn't drink soda until the last century and you can survive better without it!

Studies have shown that when people with diabetes make the change to a very low-carb, high-fat diet, that within a matter of weeks, they begin to see a drop in their fasting blood sugar, hemoglobin A1c (an indication of average glucose levels), total cholesterol, low-density lipoprotein (LDL) "bad" cholesterol and triglycerides, as well as improvement in their high-density lipoprotein (HDL) "good" cholesterol and, of course, weight loss (Dashti, 2006). Not only that, but diabetics are often able to reduce or even eliminate the need for insulin and other glucose-lowering medications, some-times within two or three weeks.

Metabolic syndrome is a common disorder in which a person has at least three of the following symptoms: abdominal obesity, high blood pressure, high-fasting blood sugar, high triglycerides, and low HDL cholesterol, and, as a result, is at higher risk of heart disease and diabetes. For people with metabolic syndrome, con-suming a lower-carb and a higher-fat diet, while eating the same number of calories, dramatically improves the signs and symptoms of this condition compared with people who eat a low-fat diet (Volek, 2009).

Possibly the most compelling evidence to date that lowering our sugar intake is a great idea for the long haul is found in a large population study, published in 2013, which clearly shows that, on average, the more sugar a person eats, the greater the likelihood is of developing diabetes (Basu, 2013). The researchers found that as sugar became more available to certain populations and its annual per capita intake increased as a result, the rate of diabetes increased proportionately.

Another important study was published in the *New England Journal of Medicine* in 2013 in which blood glucose levels were collected in 2,067 men and women as part of the Adult Changes in Thought Study. In this study, 524 people developed dementia over the follow-up period of a median of 6.8 years. The researchers found that non-diabetics with blood sugars averaging 115 milligrams per deciliter (mg/dl) over the preceding five years were more likely (1.18 to 1 odds) to have dementia than those with blood glucose of 100 mg/dl. Diabetics with average blood glucose of 190 over the preceding five years were much more likely (1.4 to 1 odds) to develop dementia than diabetics with better control and average blood glucose of 160 mg/dl (Crane, 2013).

Carbohydrate Intake: Up, Up, Up

Stephan Guyenet, Ph.D., an obesity researcher and neurobiologist, has graphed the intake in added sugar in the United States over nearly 200 years using U.S. Department of Agriculture (USDA) data and U.S. Department of Commerce reports. He found that added sugar intake increased from about 6.3 pounds per person per year in 1822 to more than 107 pounds per person per year by 1999. This does not count the sugar that naturally occurs in the foods we eat (Guyenet, 2012). In March 2014, the World Health Organization announced its recommendation that added sugar be limited to no more than 5 percent of total calories in the diet, which would be 100 calories for a 2,000-calorie diet and equivalent to about 25 grams of carbohydrate or six teaspoons of sugar. Americans typically consume three times that much added sugar.

Carbohydrate intake has fluctuated quite a bit over the last century. In the early 1900s the average person in the United States consumed about 500 grams per day of carbohydrate, but these were almost entirely in the form of whole-grain foods. Carbohydrate intake gradually declined by 25 percent to 374 grams per day by 1963, while fiber intake decreased by about 40 percent during the same time frame. Fiber intake continued to decline as ready-to-eat cereals made from refined grains came into vogue. Meanwhile, corn syrup intake and other refined carbohydrate intake increased steadily between 1963 and 1997 along with total carbohydrates, back up to 500 grams per day.

Corn syrup was almost non-existent at the beginning of the 1900s but, in 1967, high-fructose corn syrup was introduced, and by 1997 it was the sweetener of choice, and made up more than 20 percent of carbohydrates in the diet and 10 percent of daily caloric intake. Even though the percentage of fat in the diet had decreased, total energy intake had increased by more than 500 calories per day on average—nearly all of it attributable to the increase in carbohydrate intake. Between 1980 and 1997, type 2 diabetes increased by 47 percent and obesity by 80 percent, and there are few signs of the trend letting up in 2015 (Gross, 2004).

One irony of the increased use of high-fructose corn syrup is that it is often used in products called "light" foods—usually meaning they are low fat and intended to fit into the objective of a low-fat diet. However, fructose is mostly converted to fat in the form of triglycerides after it is digested and makes its way to the liver. So, it appears that the introduction of corn syrup, and especially high-fructose corn syrup, into our diets may have a great deal to do with the marked increases in obesity and diabetes in the United States over the past fifty years. Just to remind you, people with diabetes are much more likely to develop Alzheimer's disease, a type of diabetes of the brain, and other forms of dementia. Added sugars appear to play a significant role in this connection (Lakhan, 2013). Therefore, if we already have diabetes, making the change to a lower-carb and higher-fat diet and staying away from added sugar as much as possible could help us avoid some serious problems down the road. For those of us who don't have diabetes yet, we have a great opportunity to avoid it altogether.

Types of Low-Carb Diets

Ketogenic diets are low in carbohydrates and high in fat, and can be used alone or in combination with other choices to raise ketones. The strictest form of this diet, used for nearly 100 years to successfully treat severe drug-resistant childhood epilepsy, can be achieved but requires considerable motivation for the long term. Food must be carefully weighed to maintain a consistent ratio of fat to protein and carbohydrates, and a single high-carb meal can stop ketosis immediately, requiring days to return to the same levels of ketones.

The use of a strict ketogenic diet could be a viable option for highly motivated people who cannot tolerate even small amounts of coconut or MCT oil. The caregivers must be highly motivated as well, since they will be instrumental in most cases in determining what food will be on the plate. More information and help with the ketogenic diet can be found through the non-profit groups the Charlie Foundation (www.charliefoundation.org) and Matthew's Friends (www.matthewsfriends.org). More recently, this diet is under intensive investigation and shows great promise as an adjunct to treating cancer (see www.ketonutrition.org and www.ketogenic-diet-resource.com).

Less strict forms of the ketogenic diet may be more practical for most people and any measures that can be taken to reduce carbohydrates in the diet could be beneficial in the long run. Jeff S. Volek, Ph.D., and Stephen D. Phinney, M.D., have published more than

200 studies on low-carb nutrition and have helped hundreds of type 2 diabetics go into remission and come off insulin and other diabetes medications by adhering to a low-carb, high-fat diet. They present a comprehensive analysis of this work in their book *The Art and Science of Low Carbohydrate Living* (2011), and are also authors of *The New Atkins for a New You* (2010) along with Eric C. Westman, M.D. They found that keeping carbohydrate intake at 60 grams or less per day will allow most people who do not have type 2 diabetes to keep insulin levels relatively low and encourage mild ketosis.

To lose weight or to get type 2 diabetes under control, Drs. Volek and Phinney advise dropping carbohydrate intake to 20 grams per day for two weeks or longer and, after the initial period, increasing to 25 to 30 grams of carbohydrate while still losing weight, and then increasing by 5 grams at a time to find the optimal range that will help maintain weight. For most people this will be somewhere between 50 and 75 grams of carbohydrate per day (although some people may do fine with up to 125 grams per day). To further stabilize body weight after weight loss, they suggest consuming more healthy fats in the diet instead of carbohydrates to make it easier to avoid going back to old bad habits and carb craving (more on this later). This approach will not only encourage weight loss but also reduce the average blood sugar level and reduce the insulin level over time.

Another well-written and easy-to-understand version of this type of diet is *The New Atkins Made Easy* (2013) by Colette Heimowitz.

The remaining sections in this chapter will help guide you toward reducing carbohydrates to 60 grams or less per day, a reasonable amount of carbohydrate that will reduce insulin levels overall, encourage ketosis, and keep type 2 diabetes at bay for most people who are at risk—hopefully without feeling totally deprived. This is not a temporary diet but rather a permanent lifestyle change for those who are serious about avoiding these diseases and their potentially dire consequences.

DESIGNING A LOW-CARB DIET

A good place to start transitioning to a lower-carb diet is to move away from what I like to call the "convenience-food" diet and to move toward a whole-food diet. The biggest nutritional mistake we made for the first few decades of our marriage was to take the easy way out and use every excuse to eat at fast-food restaurants and to fill our pantry, refrigerator, and freezer with packaged foods. All you need to do is pop these foods in the microwave— and voila dinner is ready! Convenience foods are largely made with refined white flour, considerable added sugar, and maybe a sprinkling of vegetables; the protein content usually consists of a few pieces of real meat or chicken enhanced with soy protein, powdered milk, or powdered eggs; and the fat is often partially hydrogenated with trans fats. On top of that, convenience foods contain an abundance of chemicals to add color, flavor, and consistency, and to extend shelf life. They tasted good to us but were not good for us.

You might assume that, as a physician, I should have been knowledgeable about nutrition, but, in fact, I had only one afternoon of instruction in nutrition in four years of medical school. Sure, I had taken biochemistry and learned about the metabolism of the components of food and about the need for vitamins and signs and symptoms of vitamin deficiencies, but I learned virtually nothing else about how food can cause disease and how food can be employed to treat and prevent disease.

As I researched Alzheimer's disease and how to help Steve, it began to hit home that our diet was poor and that our poor diet could be factoring into his condition. So, while striving to learn as much as possible about good nutrition, we began the transition in early 2006 from a convenience-food diet toward a whole-food diet. We also got away from drinking soda, fruit juices that often have added sugar, and other sugary drinks, and away from eating foods with added sugars. We moved to having whole grains in smaller portions and drastically cut our intake of carbohydrates. We have both benefited in many ways by doing this. For example, my fasting blood sugar had made its way to the prediabetic range at the end of 2005. This was a serious wake-up call for me, as I was well aware of the serious complications down the road that I could expect to face if I developed diabetes. Now, for the past nine years since changing our diet, my fasting blood sugar has been stable in the normal range. After numerous yo-yo periods throughout my life of losing weight and then regaining the weight plus a few new pounds, I have managed to keep off more than forty pounds since 2006.

Out with Convenience Foods, In with Whole Foods

The cells of our bodies are extremely complex and dynamic, and we are constantly making new cells to replace old cells. What we eat will affect the quality (that is, how well they function) and the life span of the new cells we make. When we get right down to it, the main function of food is to provide fuel for our cells as well as the necessary components to make new cells and keep them running. The major components of foods—carbohydrates, protein, and fat—can all be used for fuel. These macronutrients, along with thousands of other micronutrients, are needed to make new cells by providing the required energy and the necessary building blocks. These include numerous vitamins, minerals, and antioxidants as well as a multitude of other phytonutrients.

Phytonutrients are compounds found in plants that can positively affect our health. In recent years, hundreds of phytonutrients have been discovered, and we are learning new things every day about what they do for us. Many of these phytonutrients work in conjunction with vitamins and minerals to carry out various processes in the body. Some phytonutrients prevent damage to cells, while others help keep us healthy by reducing our chances of developing infections or certain cancers. One good reason to eat a variety of colors of fresh or freshly frozen vegetables is to take in as many of these nutrients as possible every day, since they are often lost when food is canned or otherwise processed.

When we eat processed foods, not only do our bodies miss out on many of the natural substances that they need to function at their fullest potential, but we also end up consuming an abundance of chemicals that are used to enhance color and taste, inhibit the growth of bacteria and mold, and increase the shelf life of these products. The use of these food manufacturing methods has come about as a result of the huge population growth in recent history. Billions of people must be fed, and advances in technology have made it possible to mass-produce food and deliver it wherever it is needed. There is a field of science devoted to making food look and taste good (known as sensory evaluation and flavor chemistry), but this idea is often carried to extremes when the primary goal of the food manufacturer is to make money and good nutrition is thrown out the window. An excess of salt and sugar might be added for the simple reason that it will taste so good that we will want more of it. The downside of this type of thinking is that much of our food has become overly processed and laden with unnecessary additives, and potentially harmful added sugar and artificial ingredients.

From an evolutionary point of view, many of these food additives are not recognized by our cells and could be harmful. As just one example, in a November 7, 2013 news release, the FDA proclaimed that partially hydrogenated fats, which are loaded with trans fats, no longer qualified for GRAS (generally recognized as safe) status and would be phased out from foods in the United States within the next two years. In the official written statement, FDA Commissioner Margaret Hamburg said that there was no safe level of consumption of trans fat and no known benefit from consuming them, and that "further reduction in the amount of trans fat in the American diet could prevent an additional 20,000 heart attacks and 7,000 deaths from heart disease each year—a critical step in the protection of Americans' health." In the 1980s, Mary Enig, Ph.D., and other lipid biochemists were already advising the FDA that trans fats are harmful but they were ignored for many years. Finally, in 2013, the FDA began listening.

Similar concerns have been raised about high-fructose corn syrup, a common additive in packaged foods and sugary drinks discussed earlier. Concern about genetic engineering (GE) of foods such as corn, soybeans, and wheat has also been growing. The case for the genetic modification of wheat over the years and the role it may play in development of obesity, insulin resistance, and diabetes is presented in the book *Wheat Belly* (2011) by William Davis, M.D.

Making the transition to a whole-food diet may seem radical but consider that a century ago, and for millennia before that, our ancestors had little choice but to eat a whole-food diet. They did not have access to the abundance of GE, refined, and processed foods that are the norm in our modern diet. Today, we have to worry about the fertilizers used to grow vegetables, fruits, and grains, as well as the pesticides, hormones, and antibiotics taken in by the animals that are used to feed us, and the sodium nitrites and other chemicals that are used to preserve many meats, processed cheeses, and other products. We might even need to worry about the synthetic vitamins used to fortify foods like white flour and white rice, since synthetic vitamins are not the naturally occurring forms of vitamins found in whole foods. A whole-food diet is not a radical idea. What has happened to *our* food today is radical.

A whole-food diet is one in which the foods are as close to their natural form as possible; they are unrefined and minimally processed, and do not contain added ingredients such as salt and sugar. While there are exceptions and some food makers are striv-ing to produce healthier foods, in general, the foods you want to avoid with a whole-food diet are packaged cookies, crackers, pas-tries, ready-to-eat foods, sugary cereals and drinks, many breads, and snacks. These and other processed foods are usually located in the aisles at the center of the grocery store. Instead, when shopping, concentrate on the fresh produce, seafood, meat, dairy, and egg sections that make up the borders of the store. Whole foods are generally a better overall source of nutrition due to the complexity of nutrients they contain, and many of these foods are also good sources of fiber.

Examples of foods that you will want to make staples in your diet include:

- Fresh or flash-frozen vegetables and fruits
- Nuts, seeds, and legumes (beans, peanuts, and peas)
- Eggs
- Whole, unpolished grains such as whole-grain flours, brown and wild rice, quinoa, millet
- Natural oils and fats, such as olive oil, coconut oil, butter, nut butters and nut oils
- Full-fat dairy products such as milk, yogurt, eggs, and cheese from cows, goats, and sheep
- Meats, poultry, fish, and shellfish

Some packaged foods will fit into a whole-food diet and the best way to evaluate them is to look at the package ingredients closely. If the ingredients' list is limited to the foods above, and added sugar and other chemicals do not make that list, take it home by all means. If you don't recognize some of the ingredients as actual nat-ural foods, then consider putting it back on the shelf.

In 2011, the USDA changed the icon to explain its dietary guidelines from a food pyramid to a food plate (see Figure 2.1). For many years MyPyramid promoted a high-carb, low-fat diet during which time the epidemics of diabetes and obesity only worsened. And while MyPlate is a sensible improvement that divides a healthy diet into roughly four main parts—vegetables, fruits, grains, and proteins—with a glass of milk (to represent dairy) next to the plate, nonetheless, it's disappointing that more than three-fourths of the

---

GO ORGANIC, WHEN POSSIBLE

A whole-food diet is not necessarily an organic-food diet, but ideally you will want to look for organic foods as well. Here is just one good reason: Nitrogen fertilizers are generally used to grow non-organic vegetables. There is some evidence that excessive nitrates (a byproduct nitrogen fertilizers), which accumulate in many of these plants, can be metabolized in the body to toxic lipids that cross the blood-brain barrier and cause insulin resistance in the brain, hypothetically leading to diabetes and Alzheimer's disease as well (De la Monte, 2010). So, if you are going to make your diet healthier by adding more vegetables, organic is the way to go whenever possible.

Although organic foods are more available in some areas than others, more and more, even mainstream grocery stores are adding organic choices to their inventory. Likewise, meat, poultry, and fish products are now more widely available that are labeled to be grass-fed, wild-caught, or sustainably raised and free of hormones, antibiotics, sodium nitrites (used to cure meats), and other preservatives. Free-range, hormone- and antibiotic-free eggs and dairy products are also widely available. Hopefully, soon foods will also require labeling to indicate whether they contain GE organisms. This too will allow people to be more aware of the choices they are making.

plate is comprised of carbohydrates, and it contains no fat! The brain consists of at least 60 percent fat and every cell membrane in the body is made up of fats. The USDA continues to perpetuate a high-carb, low-fat diet as healthy with this icon. It fails to educate the public about the importance of healthy fats and whole grains rather than refined grains as nutrients.

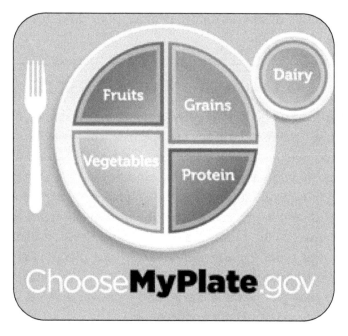

FIGURE 2.1. Where's the Fat? USDA MyPlate. Washington, DC: www.chosemyplate.gov.

Another version of the plate created by experts at the Harvard School of Public Health and Harvard Medical School is compatible with the whole-food type of diet described here. Their plate, called the Healthy Eating Plate (see Figure 2.2 on page 51), includes healthy fats and provides specific information about wise choices to fill up the plate. (The main change I would make on the Healthy Eating Plate is to add coconut oil to the list of healthy oils!)

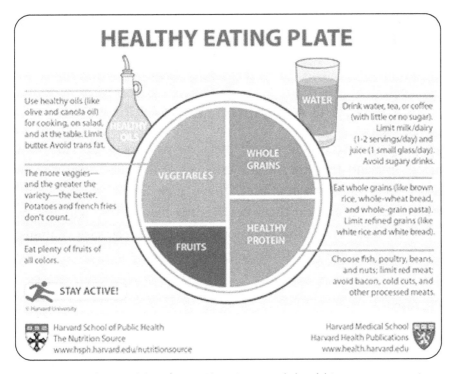

FIGURE 2.2. The Healthy Eating Plate is a much healthier representation of what we should be eating: www.hsph.harvard.edu/ nutritionsource/healthy-eating-plate.

The biggest hurdle to sticking long term with any diet is whether the foods are appealing to us. How many of us have lost weight and reached our goal on a diet that relies on packaged foods, only to return to our old way of eating and weight? If we can choose foods that we normally eat and that we like to eat, but learn to eat the right amount of these foods, which will help us avoid excess sugar intake, then we may find ourselves on the road to long-term success with achieving our goal of avoiding insulin resistance, and diabetes of the brain and other organs.

The primary goal of the diet presented here is to reduce carbohydrate intake in a way that will appeal to you. You will not be told exactly what to eat but instead you will make the choices. This is not the type of diet that will necessarily result in weight loss, but it could if you find that you are not craving carbohydrates after a while and are not eating as much food as a result.

CREATING A HEALTHY, LOW-CARB MEAL

To put together our low-carb diet, we will focus on the three macronutrients that are the cornerstones of the meals we eat: proteins, fats, and carbohydrates. If we pick a variety of quality macronutrients and eat them in a healthy balance, we will also be relatively assured that our bodies are getting the necessary vitamins, minerals, and other phytonutrients they need.

Protein

An easy way to plan any diet is to consider protein as the foundation. After figuring out how much protein we need and what specific choices we are going to make to get the right amount of it, we can then build the meal or snack around our protein choices.

Protein is an important component of every cell in the body. Protein is comprised of chains of amino acids linked by chemical bonds. Certain amino acids are considered "essential," meaning that they cannot be made by the body and must be supplied through the diet. Numerous different proteins are present in all cells. They are the building blocks of body tissues and also carry out the various functions of the cells. Certain amino acids from the breakdown of protein can be converted to glucose and used as fuel when supplies of carbohydrates and fats are low. Proteins in the diet come from eggs, milk, meats, poultry, and fish, and are also found in grains, legumes, nuts, seeds, soy, and in small amounts in vegetables and some fruits.

It is difficult to stay healthy if a person does not eat enough protein and the right kinds of protein. We need the right mix of amino acids to efficiently make the proteins our bodies need. If a couple of the essential amino acids are missing from a food, another food containing them needs to be eaten with it in order for the protein to be used efficiently. Animal proteins typically contain the full gamut of the necessary amino acids, but many vegetables, legumes, and grains do not contain much protein and, individually, may not contain all the essential amino acids. If by chance they do, they may not contain the right proportion of amino acids to efficiently make the proteins we need; consequently, specific vegetables, legumes, and grains may need to be combined at the same meal to get that full gamut of amino acids. This is why being vegan (a strict vegetarian) and staying healthy can be a challenge and should not be entered into casually. Considerable research is needed to be successful in undertaking a vegan lifestyle.

Essential as protein is, eating too much is not healthy either. Diets high in protein and fat have been widely used since physician and cardiologist Robert Atkins popularized the approach in the 1970s. In the diet's original form, unlimited protein and fat were allowed and vegetable intake was not particularly stressed. The newer, modified version of this diet limits protein intake because, when there is an excess of protein, it is not stored as such, but rather is broken down, causing some of the amino acids from the protein to be converted to sugar. Also, eating too much protein can cause complications, including development of kidney stones and gout flare-ups, and it can stress the kidneys if someone already has kidney disease. Recommendations for fat intake are also included in the newer Atkins diet plan to avoid an excess of calories overall while losing weight. See the Resources section for books on the Atkins diet.

The easiest way to figure out the minimum amount of protein you should eat in a day is to multiply $1/2$ gram times your weight in pounds or 1 gram for each kilogram (about 2 pounds) you weigh.

HOW MUCH PROTEIN?

Your weight in pounds ÷ 2 = # grams protein per day to eat

EXAMPLE: 150 pounds ÷ 2 = 75 grams per day

UPPER LIMIT: 2 × 75 grams = 150 grams

OR

Your weight in kilograms × 1 = # grams protein per day to eat

EXAMPLE: 75 kilograms × 1 = 75 grams per day

UPPER LIMIT: 2 × 75 grams = 150 grams

For example, the average person who weighs 150 pounds would want to eat at least 75 grams of protein per day to maintain lean body mass (muscle, bone and other nonfat tissues). Someone who weighs 200 pounds would take in 100 or more grams of protein per day. The upper limit of protein intake is about one and one-half to twice that much—about 150 grams for that 150-pound person would be the max to shoot for. There is no particular advantage to eating more protein than that unless you are an avid bodybuilder. Keeping it simple, each gram of protein provides about 4 calories. So, 100 grams of protein would provide about 400 calories in your daily diet.

Protein is digested slowly and doesn't cause a spike in insulin. Because of this, including some protein with each meal and snack can help you last longer in between without feeling hungry. Eating an ounce or two of cheese (about 100 to 200 calories), which contains no carbohydrates, will keep you happy a lot longer and without causing a spike in insulin than a high-carb snack (such as an energy bar or a glass of orange juice), which will spike your insulin and likely make you want more of the same not long after.

Table 2.1 on page 55 will help you figure out what to eat to get enough protein every day. To make it simple, the number of grams is rounded and could be plus or minus 1 gram.

TABLE 2.1. PROTEIN CONTENT OF SOME COMMON FOODS

# Grams protein per serving (+/− 1 gram)	Proteins; Food and serving size
25	3 ounces of beef, pork, poultry, lamb, or tuna, cooked; 1 cup full-fat cottage cheese or ricotta
21	3 ounces of most fish (except tuna and cod) or lobster, cooked; 1 cup green soybeans, boiled
15	3 ounces cod, crab, or shrimp; 1 cup plain full-fat Greek yogurt
8	2 tablespoons peanut or almond butter
7	1 ounce hard cheese
6	1 egg; 8 ounces of full-fat cow's, goat's or sheep's milk; 1 ounce soft cheese, such as Brie or blue cheese; 1 to $1^{1}/_{2}$ ounces nuts; $^{1}/_{2}$ cup most beans
3	3 slices nitrite-, preservative-, hormone-, antibiotic-free bacon
2 or less	$^{1}/_{2}$ cup most vegetables or 1 cup leafy green vegetables, cooked; $^{1}/_{3}$ cup undiluted coconut milk or 1 ounce grated coconut
0–1	Nearly all fruits, 1 medium or typical serving

Note: The composition of most common whole and processed foods, including grams of protein, can be found on the USDA website at ndb.nal.usda.gov/ndb/search.

For instance, if you weigh 150 pounds and engage in an average amount of exercise, you would want to eat a minimum of 75 grams of protein per day. Your protein choices over the course of the day could be:

- Three eggs and 1 ounce of grated cheese with breakfast
- 3 ounces of turkey for lunch
- 3 ounces of chicken for dinner
- 1 ounce of nuts and one ounce of cheese for snacks

Your meals will, of course, include carbohydrates and fats as well. If you are a very active muscular 150-pound person, you could take more and perhaps even double the portion sizes of each of these protein food items. Since there is not much protein in most vegetables, just consider the protein from these as a bonus for our purposes here. Most fruits have 1 gram or less per serving.

Fats

Now let's talk about fats (technically called lipids). These include solid fats and liquid oils—substances that usually do not dissolve in water.

In the diet, fat comes in several forms, including saturated, monounsaturated, and polyunsaturated. Most fats and oils are combinations of two, or even all three, of these forms. They are comprised of fatty acids that are bound with a glycerol molecule to make triglycerides.

In the body, fat insulates and protects the muscles and internal organs and acts as a storage form of energy. It is a major component of every cell membrane. It makes up 60 to 70 percent of the brain (along with an abundance of cholesterol, which supports the structure of cell membranes and the delicate network of brain cells), and is involved in communication between brain cells, as well as many other important functions. In addition, hormones and many other important substances are derived from fatty acids, and many substances are stored in fat.

Two types of fatty acids that are essential for health and that cannot be made by the body, and therefore must be obtained from the diet, are alpha-linolenic acid (an omega-3 fatty acid) and alpha-linoleic acid (an omega-6 fatty acid). The body does not need much of these fatty acids compared to the total amount of daily fat intake, but they need to be in balance. One huge problem with the American diet is that, due to the amount and types of vegetable oils in home-cooked and restaurant food, we tend to eat an overabundance of omega-6 fats and not enough omega-3 fats. Why this is a problem and how much omega-3 and omega-6 fats we should eat is addressed in the inset on page 81. Since omega-3 fat is a relatively small component of our overall fat intake (about 1 gram per day or less) and the omega-6 requirement (between 1 and 4 grams), we will not factor these into the calculation of how much fat to consume except to stress that it is important to include these essential fatty acids in the overall diet.

Few topics create more controversy in the field of nutrition than a discussion about how much fat to eat and what constitutes a good or bad fat. U.S. government recommendations for nutrition are updated every five years in a document titled *Dietary Guidelines for Americans,* with the most recent update in 2010. An advisory group of nutrition experts develop these recommendations. So, how much fat should we consume?

HOW MUCH FAT?

The recommendation for fat intake since the 2005 edition comes from guidelines put forth by the Institute of Medicine (IOM), which advises that fat intake for adults should be between 20 and 35 percent of total calories. Twenty percent is considered the minimum amount of fat needed to ensure an adequate intake of calories, essential fatty acids, and fat-soluble vitamins.

The list of references used by the IOM to reach these conclusions is extensive. However, in their comprehensive publication *Dietary Reference Intakes for Energy, Carbohydrate, Fiber, Fat, Fatty Acids, Cholesterol, Protein, and Amino Acids,* the IOM acknowledges under the "Research Recommendations" regarding fat consumption that "randomized and blinded long-term (greater than one year) studies are needed on the effect of dietary fat versus carbo-hydrate on body fatness," and regarding saturated fats that "fur-ther examination of intakes at which significant risk of chronic diseases can occur is needed" (IOM, 2005).

The *Dietary Guidelines for Americans, 2010* also advises that liquid fats should be chosen over solid fats (solid at room tempera-ture) as much as possible, and that saturated fat intake should be less than 10 percent of the total fat intake. These recommendations are based on the ideas that we should be eating a low-fat diet and that saturated fat is bad. The guidelines contain a chart showing the relative proportions of saturated fat, monounsaturated fat, and polyunsaturated fat but failing to differentiate between medium-chain saturated fats, which behave very differently than long-chain saturated fats. Both coconut oil and palm kernel oil contain a larger proportion of medium-chain saturated fats than long-chain ones (as discussed in Chapter 3), so the chart in the *Dietary Guidelines for Americans, 2010* and other comments made about these two oils are misleading in this respect.

If we go with the upper limit of 35 percent of total calories for fat intake according to the *Dietary Guidelines,* which translates to 78 grams of a 2,000-calorie diet, we can easily accommodate 3 to 4 tablespoons or more of coconut oil into the diet at 14 grams per tablespoon. As we reduce carbohydrates in the diet, we can allow for higher fat intake to compensate for the difference in calories.

As a society, we have been programmed for decades to fear eat-ing fat. Over the last sixty or so years, with much stress on eating a low-fat diet, it would seem that all-natural fats are bad and that synthetic fats like Crisco and margarines (most of which are pre-pared with partially hydrogenated man-made fats and loaded with unnatural trans fats) are what we should be eating to avoid heart disease. Folks middle age and older will likely remember mar-garines advertised extensively as heart healthy to use in place of butter. People who took low-fat-diet message to heart (pun intended) and switched from butter and other animal fats that our ancestors consumed for eons to these poor substitutes, naturally compensated for the loss of fat calories by greatly increasing their intake of carbohydrates, which we now know has resulted in an abundance of health issues.

As an aside, the *Dietary Guidelines for Americans, 2010* also puts forth a recommendation that at least half of grains be consumed as whole grains, allowing that the other half can be comprised of refined grains, which have been stripped of fiber and other important nutrients and fortified with supplemental vitamins. Given that there is no dietary need for refined grains and that they may actually be detrimental to our health, it is perplexing that this advisory group doesn't go all the way in recommending that we should strive to eat all grain as whole grains in our diets.

Furthermore, in the *Dietary Guidelines for Americans, 2010,* there is a table showing that, in the late 1970s, 15 percent of adults were obese. By the early 1990s, this number had jumped to 25 percent and, by 2008, 34 percent of adults were considered obese. The increase corresponds to the exact time frame in which the U.S. government published recommendations and engaged in a highly publicized campaign encouraging Americans to consume a low-fat diet. That table is followed by another table, this one on the top twenty-five sources of calories among Americans, ages two and older. The table shows that Americans consume an inordinate amount of carbohydrate: the top four foods in children, ages two through eighteen, are grain-based desserts, pizza, soda/energy/sports drinks, and yeast breads; the top four foods in adults are grain-based desserts, yeast breads, chicken and chicken-mixed dishes (which include breaded and fried chicken), and soda/energy/sports drinks. Alcoholic beverages, pizza, tortillas/burritos/tacos, and pasta and pasta dishes ranked numbers five through eight for adults. Vegetables and whole fruits (as opposed to fruit juice) did not make the top twenty-five sources of calories for children or adults.

Fat is a very dense form of energy. It supplies about 9 calories per gram, compared to just over 4 calories per gram of either carbohydrate or protein. There is a limit to how much protein we should eat, as you learned earlier. But to provide enough energy to keep our bodies running, if we take fat out of the equation, we need to take in more than twice as much carbohydrate to get the same number of calories. This means that for a single tablespoon or 14 grams of fat we remove from the diet, we would need to eat almost 32 grams of carbohydrates. (We will see in the upcoming section on Carbohydrates why that creates a dilemma for us.)

We need to overcome our fear of eating fat. Unless we eat excess calories in general, eating fat will not cause us to become fatter. Not only that, but coconut oil and saturated fat do not "clog" arteries. Much has been learned in the field of lipid biochemistry since this idea was originated based on flawed science and, in spite of a myriad of studies proving otherwise, this is a myth that won't die easily. Biochemist Beverly Teter has studied fats and oils for decades, including coconut oil, and is coauthor with cardiologist Stephen Sinatra and others of an important article that appeared in the the the *Journal of the American College of Nutrition* titled, "The Saturated Fat, Cholesterol, and Statin Controversy: A Commentary" (Sinatra, 2014). This article reviews the history of the prevailing myths and the important studies that refute them, as well as their opinions of which fats to eat and which to avoid. Coconut oil is among the healthy fats they discuss. Specifically, they mention lauric acid, a medium-chain triglyceride that makes up about half of coconut oil and that, as mentioned earlier, has antimicrobial properties, which support the immune system and, therefore, help fight many types of infection. They also point out that lard or animal fat per se are not a problem, but rather the toxins that accumulate in the fat of animals, such as cattle, that are fed with GE foods, which are generally grown with potentially harmful pesticides and insecticides, and are also fed hormones and antibiotics. Could it be that it is the chemicals found in beef, and/or the glycation that occurs when it is grilled, that are harmful and not so much the actual meat itself? Following are the fats that you will want to keep in your diet and those you may want to avoid or minimize.

Good fats

- Coconut oil

- Fat in dark chocolate

- Fats in mixed nuts, olives, and avocados

- Fatty fish and fish oil (certified to be mercury-free)

- Olive, sunflower, and canola oils (high in monounsaturated fats)

- Organic cow-, sheep- and goat-milk fats, including butter

- Organic lard and fat from grass-fed/cage-free or organically fed animals

Bad fats

- Corn oil (high in omega-6 fats)*

- Fat from GE-fed livestock (may contain pesticides and insecticides)

- Lard from GE-fed livestock (may contain pesticides and insecticides)

- Partially hydrogenated margarines (contains trans fats)

- Partially hydrogenated solid shortenings (contains trans fats)

- Safflower oil (high in omega-6 fats)*

- Soybean oil (high in omega-6 fats)*

* Note: These oils are high in omega-6 fats and have minimal omega-3; minimize their use.

If we include many of the whole foods mentioned earlier and in the list of good fats above, we will already be getting some healthy fat in our diet. These include meats, poultry, fish, eggs, nuts, olives, avocados, and full-fat dairy products from cows, goats, and sheep. Table 2.2 lists the gram content of these and other common fats.

# Net grams fat per serving (+/- 0.5 to 1 gram)	Fats; Food and Servings
32	1 cup full-fat ricotta
30	1 medium avocado
22	1 cup plain full-fat Greek yogurt
21	1 ounce macadamia nuts
17–20	1 ounce Brazil nuts, pecans, or walnuts; 2 tablespoons almond butter; 2 tablespoons peanut butter; 1 cup full-fat sheep's milk; $1/3$ cup grated, unsweetened coconut
15–16	1 ounce almonds or peanuts; 2 x 2 x $1/2$-inch piece raw coconut meat
13–14	1 ounce cashews or pistachios; 1 tablespoon coconut oil, MCT oil, palm kernel oil, all other oils, and lard
12	3-ounce serving fattier cuts of beef, pork and lamb, trimmed and roasted
11	1 tablespoon mayonnaise; 1 tablespoon butter; 1 cup green soybeans, boiled
10	1 cup full-fat goat's milk; 3 ounces farm-raised salmon, cooked
9	1 ounce hard cheese; 1 cup plain full-fat yogurt (not Greek); $1/2$ cup granola
8	1 cup full-fat cow's milk; 1 ounce soft cheese, such as Brie or blue
6–7	3 ounces leaner cuts of beef, pork and lamb, trimmed and roasted; 3 ounces turkey or chicken dark meat, roasted; 3 ounces wild salmon, cooked
5	1 tablespoon cream 1 cup of many cold cereals 1 large raw egg

TABLE 2.2. FAT CONTENT OF SOME COMMON FOODS

# Net grams fat per serving (+/- 0.5 to 1 gram)	Fats; Food and Servings
4	1 small egg
3	3 ounces turkey or chicken white meat, roasted
	1 cup cooked old-fashioned rolled oats
	1 tablespoon undiluted coconut milk
2-2.5	1 ounce olives
	1 tablespoon sour cream
1.5	1 tablespoon half-and-half
	1 cup cooked long-grain brown rice
1	3 ounces tuna or crab
	1 slice most white and whole-wheat bread
<1	3 ounces cod, lobster, shrimp or sole
	$1/2$ cup most legumes (beans)
	1 serving of nearly all fresh fruits and vegetables (except avocados and olives)
	$1/2$ cup refined white flour
	1 cup cooked white rice
	1 medium potato, baked
	1 medium sweet potato, baked
	1 large ($6^1/_2$-inch diameter) whole-wheat pita
	1 cup fruit or vegetable juice
	1 cup cooked cream of rice or wheat cereal
	1 cup of low-fat cold cereal
0	1 tablespoon agave, corn syrup, honey, table sugar,

Source: *The Nutribase Complete Book of Food Counts* (Avery 2001) and package nutrient labels.

Note: The composition of most common whole and processed foods, including grams of fat, can be found on the USDA website at ndb.nal.usda.gov/ndb/search.

Carbohydrates

Carbohydrates include simple sugars and more complex starches, and are also known as saccharides (mono-, di-, oligo- and polysaccharides depending on how many saccharides are strung together). Carbohydrates can be used for fuel (energy), usually in the form of glucose, and the excess can be stored for future use as glycogen, mostly in the muscles and the liver. Carbohydrates are also part of our DNA and RNA (molecules that encode and translate the genetic code) and a myriad of other biochemical reactions in the body. All the needed carbohydrates can be made from other substances in the body; none are considered "essential," meaning that the body does not need to acquire any specific carbohydrate from a food source. Fiber is an indigestible form of carbohydrate. Ultimately, most carbohydrates in the diet come from plant foods, and milk and milk products.

It is extremely difficult and, perhaps even unwise, to try to completely eliminate carbohydrates from the diet. However, there are many steps we can take to avoid overdoing carbohydrates and to make wiser choices that will help us avoid the repeated spikes in insulin levels that could lead us down the path to insulin resistance, diabetes, and even dementia. So, for those who would like to maintain higher ketone levels while taking coconut oil, the goal in this section is to become familiar with the carbohydrate content of foods and to aim for a total carbohydrate intake of 60 grams or less per day. A limit of 60 grams of carbohydrate per day will keep insulin levels under control and will also support ketosis for most people. Some people with type 2 diabetes may need to cut their carbohydrate intake even more to get the most benefit.

To give you a basic idea of where to start with counting carbohydrates, Table 2.3 on page 66 provides the approximate carbohydrate content in typical servings of common foods. Because fiber does not impact insulin levels, it is subtracted from the total amount of carbohydrate. You may quickly notice that many of the

HOW MUCH CARBOHYDRATE?

Reducing carbohydrate intake to 60 grams or less per day, is a reasonable amount of carbohydrate that will reduce insulin levels overall, encourage ketosis, and keep type 2 diabetes at bay for most people who are at risk. People who have type 2 diabetes already, and are on insulin or other diabetes medications, can expect to reduce or even get off those medications after several weeks by adhering to an even lower carbohydrate diet that is between 20 and 25 grams per day to start. After several months, gradually increasing this intake to 40 to 50 grams per day will keep most diabetics in remission.

higher-carb items on the list are foods made with flour—be it white or whole wheat—such as bagels, muffins, noodles, and pasta. Rice and white potatoes are also high on the list. One high-carb surprise included on this list to make a point is a nutritional supplement often used by elderly people to maintain their weight called Ensure Plus. This drink contains 50 grams of carbohydrate per serving, all from sugar or corn maltodextrin (a synthetic molecule linking glucose together in chains) and no fiber. About three-quarters of older people are diabetic or prediabetic, so marketing such high-carb foods to the elderly may not be such a good idea.

Milk and fruits tend to be in the moderate carbohydrate range. While the calories we get from vegetables are mainly from carbohydrates, vegetables are mostly water, contain fiber, and are not high in carbohydrates. Based on typical serving sizes, most vegetables (except peas and corn) and nuts are in the low-carb range at 2 or fewer grams per serving. Eggs, shellfish, cheeses, butter, and cream have minimal carbohydrates, and oils, including coconut oil, as well as meats, fish, and poultry have virtually none. So, this gives you an idea of which foods you might want to cut back on and those you might want to target when putting together your meals.

TABLE 2.3. CARBOHYDRATE CONTENT OF SOME COMMON FOODS

# NET GRAMS CARBOHYDRATE* PER SERVING (+/- 1 GRAM)	CARBOHYDRATES (SUGARS AND STARCHES); FOOD AND SERVINGS
74	1 Dunkin' Donuts bagel
55 to 85	1 Dunkin' Donuts muffin
51	1 medium potato (flesh and skin), baked
50	2 glazed doughnuts
	8 ounces Ensure Plus Nutrition Shake
42	$1/_2$ cup white flour
41	12-ounce can Coca-Cola Classic
	1 cup cooked long-grain brown or white rice
40	$1/_2$ cup whole-wheat flour
	1 cup cooked white or whole-wheat egg noodles or pasta
	8 ounces yogurt with fruit on bottom
38	3 (4-inch diameter) pancakes
36	1 cup most legumes (beans) (except green string beans)
32	1 cup cooked corn
30	1 large ($6 1/_2$-inch diameter) whole-wheat pita
28	$1/_2$ cup granola
	1 medium sweet potato, baked
	$1/_4$ cup raisins
26	1 medium banana
	1 cup cooked regular (not instant) oatmeal, cream of rice or wheat cereal
25	8 ounces orange juice
	1 cup of many cold cereals
22	2 slices, most white or whole-wheat bread

22 (cont.)	1 medium pear
	1 cup peas, boiled
	1 cup acorn squash, baked
17	1 medium apple
	1 cup plain full-fat yogurt (not Greek)
15	1 tablespoon agave (honey-like syrup made from plants), corn syrup, or honey
14	8 ounces Gatorade Sports Drink 14
	$^1/_2$ cup grapes
13	1 medium nectarine
12	1 tablespoon table sugar
	1 cup full-fat cow's or goat's milk
	1 medium orange
	1 cup plain full-fat Greek yogurt
	$^1/_2$ cup blueberries
10	8 ounces tomato juice or V-8 Vegetable Juice
7–9	1 medium peach or fig
	$^1/_2$ medium grapefruit
	1 cup halved strawberries
	1 ounce cashews
5–6	1 cup full-fat cottage cheese or ricotta
	$^1/_2$ cup blackberries
	$^1/_2$ cup sliced beets
	$^1/_2$ cup boiled onions
	1 cup cherry tomatoes or 1 medium tomato
	1 whole lime or lemon
2–4	1 medium apricot
	$^1/_2$ cup raspberries
	1 medium avocado

# Net grams carbohydrate* per serving (+/– 1 gram)	Carbohydrates (Sugars and Starches); Food and servings
2–4 (cont.)	4 asparagus spears
	1 ounce almonds, Brazil nuts, macadamias, peanuts, and walnuts
	$1/_2$ cup broccoli or cauliflower, cooked
	$1/_2$ cup green beans (string or snap beans) or turnips, cooked
	$1/_2$ cup bell or sweet peppers, cooked
	1 cup boiled, chopped kale or other dark leafy greens
	1 cup chopped cucumber or celery
	3 ounces lobster
	1 tablespoon catsup or sweet relish
0–1	1 whole raw egg
	1 ounce hard or semi-soft cheese
	3 ounces shrimp or crab
	1 tablespoon butter, cream, half-and-half, sour cream
	1 cup of most lettuces, spinach, other leafy greens, and cabbages
	1 medium carrot or radish
	1 cup yellow or zucchini squash, cooked
	1 ounce olives
	1 ounce pecans or pistachios
	1 tablespoon mayonnaise, mustard, dill relish, vinegar
0	Beef, fish, lamb, pork, poultry,
	Coconut oil, MCT oil, all other oils, butter, and lard

* Net grams of carbohydrates = Total grams minus grams of fiber

Source: *The Nutribase Complete Book of Food Counts* (Avery, 2001) and package nutrient labels.

Note: The composition of most common whole and processed foods, including grams of carbohydrates, can be found on the USDA website at ndb.nal.usda.gov/ndb/search.

Keeping in mind that we are planning to keep our carbohydrate intake at 60 grams per day or less, you will quickly notice that the usual serving sizes of some foods will put us over the top in short order. Perhaps by having a greater awareness of how many carbohydrates are in our favorite foods, we can find a way to adjust our diet to keep many of the foods we enjoy but just eat less of them or better yet to eat them only occasionally.

PUTTING IT ALL TOGETHER: A ONE-DAY SAMPLE MENU

Now, to get started we will put together a few different breakfast meals with similar calorie counts for comparison to get an idea of what we might decide *not* to do in the future versus some better choices. For example, many of us grew up with the notion that we should drink a glass of orange juice for breakfast, but a single 8-ounce glass of orange juice contains 25 grams of carbohydrate, almost half of our 60-carb daily limit. Even worse, the 12-ounce can of Coca-Cola Classic that many people jolt themselves awake with has 41 grams of pure sucrose sugar, which is roughly half glucose and half fructose. Are there better choices that might make us just as happy but that don't use up our daily carbohydrate allowance first thing in the morning?

Breakfast

Here are several breakfast combinations between 540 and 600 calories, each with a very different amount of carbohydrates. For breakfast you could choose from the following:

MEAL #1 HIGH IN CARBOHYDRATES

8 ounces of orange juice

+ 1$^1/_2$ cups cold cereal

+ 8 ounces milk

+ 1 slice toast with 1 pat margarine and covered with jelly

+ coffee with 1 tablespoon flavored coffee creamer

= a whopping 90 grams CARBS + only 10 grams PROTEIN
(and about 600 calories) and likely contains partially hydrogenated
fat in the margarine and creamer that we want to avoid.

This meal has already surpassed our daily carbohydrate maximum and does not
contain much protein. Your insulin will surge and you will probably be hungry
well before lunch.

OR

MEAL #2 LOWER IN CARBOHYDRATES

1 cup plain, full-fat Greek yogurt
(sweetened with liquid stevia to taste, if desired)

+ $^1/_2$ cup halved strawberries

+ 1 tablespoon sliced almonds

+ 5 ounces Thin-Style Coconut Milk (recipe on page 142)

+ coffee with 1 tablespoon real cream

= 18 grams CARBS and 20 grams PROTEIN (about 540 calories)

This meal contains nearly twice as much protein and about one-quarter the
carbohydrates of Meal #1 and no unnatural trans fat. Your insulin level will
rise somewhat but much lower and you will be satisfied much longer due to
the higher protein content of the meal.

OR

MEAL #3 EVEN LOWER IN CARBOHYDRATES

3-egg omelet with 1-ounce shredded cheddar cheese

+ 6 cherry tomatoes cut in half

+ 6 Kalamata olives, cooked in a skillet with
1 or more tablespoons coconut oil

+ 3 slices nitrite-, preservative-, hormone-, antibiotic-free bacon

+ coffee with 1 tablespoon real cream

= 9 CARBS + 24 grams PROTEIN (about 610 calories)

This meal has less than one-tenth the carbohydrates as Meal #1 and more than twice the protein for about the same number of calories.

To find out for yourself which meal will hold you longer, consider trying these three meals on three different days and keep a record of how much time elapses before you begin to feel hungry again. Also, when you do get hungry, think about whether you are longing for something sweet. Chances are, that with the second or third meal, you will last longer and you will not be thinking as much about sugar. After just a week or two of eating a lower-carb diet, if you have been a carboholic up to this point, your mindset could change from constantly thinking about the next meal and craving sugar to feeling satisfied for hours and being remarkably happy to eat healthy proteins, vegetables, whole grains, and fats at the next meal.

Does this mean we have to give up everything we like to eat? No more bread or cereal? Sounds pretty boring. Let's think about this for a minute. One trend in recent years, with the American diet in particular, is a hefty increase in portion sizes. We have been super-sized along with this trend as a result. What if we reversed this trend and started thinking about just eating less of the things we like? We can develop a new strategy by thinking it through and planning more carefully.

For example, if you are trying to stay under 60 grams and choose the 9-carb breakfast (Meal #3), you still have about 50 carbs to distribute with the other meals and snacks throughout the day. Do you really have to have two slices of bread to make a sandwich at lunchtime, or could you do it with one, or maybe even find a high-fiber, low-carb wrap to make our sandwich with? Do you need to eat a whole cup of cooked white rice with dinner, which contains 53 grams of carbohydrates, or could you learn to be just as happy with a half cup or even a quarter cup tossed with some coconut oil to make the meal a little more filling? Better yet, could you choose whole-grain rice instead, which contains the same number of carbohydrates, but an abundance of additional nutrients? Instead of a mountain of mashed potatoes covered with gravy, couldn't you choose to have a small mound mixed with a tablespoon of butter or coconut oil and a much-lower carb salad with one of the simple MCT and coconut oil salad dressings in Chapter 5? Instead of one-half cup of granola with 28 grams of carbohydrates as the centerpiece of your breakfast, could you have one-half cup of plain, full-fat Greek yogurt, sweetened with stevia and topped with a sprinkle of granola and some sliced almonds, for less than half as many carbs?

It is all about choices. The more we start thinking this way and find a compromise between what we think we want and what we truly need, the better off we will be in the long run. Ultimately, it is our longevity and quality of life that matters to us and to our families.

I have had a number of people tell me that one of the biggest plusses they have experienced after changing over to a lower-carb, higher-fat diet is that they just feel better. They have more energy, they don't tire as easily, and they often sleep better as well. I can tell you from experience that a couple of holiday seasons ago when I relapsed for a few days into carb overload, I felt more sluggish and tired, my stomach was very unhappy with indigestion and heartburn, and I was thinking way too much about chocolate. This experience was a harsh reminder of how I felt most days for many years when I lived on a convenience-food diet and was prediabetic, had osteoporosis and an enlarged heart, and was more than forty pounds heavier. I decided not to wait until New Year's Day to stop eating this way and, within a day or two of resuming my low-carb diet, returned to a healthier and happier place. Most of us won't be perfect and may choose to treat ourselves here and there, but any steps we can take to reduce sugar will be beneficial in the long run. The more consistent we are, the more benefit we will likely experience. So, let's go back to the day with the 9-gram carb breakfast. What can you do with the other 51 grams of your daily carbohydrate allowance? You could have at least five servings of most vegetables and add only 10 to 15 grams of non-fiber carbohydrate. With the remaining carbohydrates, you could have a piece of fruit and a half-cup of whole-grain pasta or two slices of whole-grain bread with lunch and dinner.

Table 2.4 below provides the gram content for smaller portions of some higher-carb choices.

TABLE 2.4. SOME HIGH-CARB FOODS REDUCED TO SMALLER PORTIONS

# NET GRAMS CARBOHYDRATE PER SERVING (+/− 1 GRAM)	CARBOHYDRATES; FOOD AND SERVING SIZE
30	1 medium (3-inch diameter) whole-grain bagel
25	$1/2$ medium baked potato (flesh and skin)
	1 glazed doughnut (only if you must!)
20	$1/2$ cup cooked whole-wheat egg noodles or pasta
	$1/2$ cup most legumes (beans, except green string beans)
	$1/2$ cup long-grain brown or white rice, cooked
15	$1/2$ large ($6^1/2$-inch diameter) whole-wheat pita
	$1/2$ medium (3-inch diameter) whole-grain bagel

# NET GRAMS CARBOHYDRATE PER SERVING (+/– 1 GRAM)	CARBOHYDRATES; FOOD AND SERVING SIZE
14	3 cups microwave popcorn
	$1/4$ cup granola
	$1/2$ medium sweet potato, flesh only
13	$1/2$ medium banana
	4 ounces orange juice
	$1/2$ cup cooked regular (not instant) cream of wheat cereal
12	1 medium orange
	$1/2$ cup baked potato, flesh only
	1 (4-inch diameter) pancake
11	1 (1-ounce) slice whole-wheat bread
10	$1/4$ cup long-grain brown rice, cooked
	$1/2$ medium pear
9	$1/4$ cup cooked corn
	1 medium peach
	$1/2$ medium apple
	$1/2$ cup plain, full-fat yogurt (not Greek)
7	$1/2$ cup boiled peas
6	$1/2$ cup plain, full-fat Greek yogurt
4	$1/2$ cup halved strawberries
3	$1/2$ cup raspberries
	$1/2$ cup ricotta or cottage cheese

With good planning, if you really cannot do without a bagel now and then, you can have a medium bagel or even a half a medium bagel on a given day, eat more protein to make the meal last longer, and then make lower-carb choices for the other meals and snacks. It's all about thinking ahead. Table 2.4 with its smaller portion sizes is just a sampling of the possibilities. You can read labels to look at the number of grams of carbohydrate and then measure out a portion size that will fit the bill. Make a list of your own favorite foods to keep as a reference, look up the carbohydrate content, and figure out portion sizes that will make you happy and that will keep your total-carb intake under control.

When you go to a restaurant, skip the bread (or at least go light on it) and ask for another side of vegetables instead of the pasta or mashed potatoes. If you feel you would like dessert, a square or two of dark chocolate (85 percent or higher) is a good choice. An occasional restaurant dessert won't likely do you in for good, but consider going for a mini- or child-size dessert or splitting a larger dessert with others at the table. Some savvy food creators are tuning into the low-carb movement and coming up with some tasty treats that don't contain an abundance of chemical additives. Or make your own tasty treats (see Chapter 5) like coconut "fudge" by combining half coconut oil and half dark chocolate—it's a great way to get some coconut oil and satisfy a sweet tooth at the same time without an excess of carbohydrate.

Lunch, Dinner, and Snacks

Suppose we opt to begin our day with the 9-gram breakfast. Now, let's go back to the choices from page 55 for 75 grams of protein, and add the fat and some additional carbohydrates to plan a sample menu for the whole day:

BREAKFAST

Three-egg omelet with 1 ounce of shredded cheese,
6 halved cherry tomatoes, and 6 Kalamata olives

1 tablespoon coconut oil for cooking the omelet

3 slices nitrite-free, preservative-free, hormone-free, antibiotic-free bacon

Coffee with 1 tablespoon real cream

LUNCH

3 ounces of turkey in a high-fiber, low-carb spinach wrap
with lettuce, tomatoes, and onions

Dressing for the wrap made of 1 tablespoon
MCT and Coconut Oil 4:3 Mixture* and
1 tablespoon ranch-style dressing

One medium orange

DINNER

3 ounces of Sybil's Coconut Chicken Tenders*

Cooked in 2 tablespoons coconut oil

Chopped Greek Salad* with one tablespoon olive oil,
lemon and Greek spice mix

SNACKS

$1/2$ cup coconut milk

Small handful of nuts, any type

One ounce of cheese

* Note: See Chapter 5 for recipes.

This all-day meal plan will provide about 91 grams of protein,
60 grams of carbohydrates, and the equivalent of five tablespoons
of coconut oil, as well as some healthy olive oil and fats that naturally occur in the protein foods—for a total of about 2,000 calories.
If you double all the protein in these meals, your total calorie count
will still come up to less than 2,400 calories a day.

OTHER CONSIDERATIONS

Until now, we have been talking about making some changes in the foods we eat, but here are some other substances we consume that we should consider or reconsider as well.

Consider Going Gluten-Free

Go yet another step further and reduce or, better yet, remove gluten from your diet. There is mounting evidence that diets high in gluten (a protein that helps foods maintain their shape) may contribute to development of insulin resistance and ultimately Alzheimer's, as discussed in detail in *Grain Brain* (2013) by David Perlmutter, a Florida neurologist whose own father, a neurosurgeon, suffers from Alzheimer's. Eliminating gluten will effectively remove a substantial amount of carbohydrates from the diet. Wheat is the most common source of gluten, but it turns up in many other grains, including barley, rye, and triticale, and in unexpected places, for example, as an additive that provides a certain consistency in processed foods, such as cereals and ice cream, and also in many condiments like mayonnaise and ketchup. The FDA does not require that gluten is listed as "gluten" on food labels and may be called other names such as flour, emulsifier, food starch, modified food starch, dextrin, maltodextrin, and vegetable gum. Dr. Perlmutter joins a growing number of experts who agree that the low-fat diet (which usually leads to a high-carb intake) should be replaced with a diet higher in healthy fats and lower in carbohydrates.

Wheat has been greatly modified over the years and the effect of eating it is to substantially raise insulin levels, whether as refined or whole-grain wheat flour. According to cardiologist William Davis in his book *Wheat Belly* (2014), there is virtually no wheat readily available in the United States today that has not been genetically engineered, and eating it contributes to accumulation of excessive fat around abdominal organs.

Therefore, give some consideration to greatly reducing or eliminating gluten and wheat (durum, einkorn, emmer, farina, farro, kamut, spelt) from the diet. If gluten is contributing to brain fog or even more serious symptoms, it will not take long to notice a difference—a matter of weeks, according to Dr. Perlmutter. Many whole grains are available that are not wheat and have no gluten, including amaranth, arrowroot, buckwheat, chia, corn, millet, potato, quinoa, rice, rolled or steel-cut oats (if labeled gluten-free), sorghum, soy, tapioca, and teff. Coconut flour and flours made from some of these grains can be used to make breads, pancakes, and other tasty gluten-free foods.

Consider Supplements a Backup to Healthy Diet

I know of many people who take a huge number of different supplements to try to undo the damage from Alzheimer's, Parkinson's, or some other disease yet continue to eat an overly processed diet, stripped of nutrients and laden with sugar, chemical additives, and partially hydrogenated fats with trans fats. It makes good sense to try to provide ourselves with nutrients that our bodies will recognize and use the way evolution has programmed us to use them. While certain supplements, such as omega-3 fatty acids, may help us in the fight against disease, supplements alone are not able to overcome the ongoing damage that we inflict on ourselves by continuing to consume a convenience-food diet.

I have also spoken with many caregivers who provide their loved ones with an abundance of different supplements but pay little attention to their diet. They cannot be convinced how important it is for their loved ones to stop drinking soda or binging on other sugary, highly processed foods that promote insulin resistance. One difficult concern for caregivers of those with Alzheimer's or Parkinson's is how much we should try to control their diet. As caregivers, chances are we are buying and bringing home the groceries. Should we bring home foods that will help them reduce their carbohydrate intake and deprive them of the sweets that they love, or is it kinder to let them enjoy this type of diet if it seems to make them happy? I don't have the answer to that question, except to say that there is enough evidence that a whole-food, low-carb diet could buy some extra years and probably better quality years (Martinez-Lapiscina, 2013). If someone is in an early to moderate stage of one of these diseases, such a diet is strongly worth considering.

Many important nutrients are not absorbed into the body unless fat is in the meal. For instance, vitamins A, D, and E are fat-soluble vitamins, which means that unless they are in an oil-based substance or at least are emulsified so they can mix with water, they will not be absorbed. It may be pointless to try to get your daily requirement of these vitamins in the form of a dry pill. It is more beneficial to get these vitamins in an oil-based product, and even better, in an actual food in which they naturally occur, such as cod liver oil, full-fat dairy products, and eggs.

Many people who research online are aware that toxicity from aluminum, cadmium, lead, and mercury may contribute in some way to Alzheimer's disease. Some other metals that are needed in small amounts to carry out normal cell functions can accumulate in the brain and cause damage as well when taken in excessive amounts, including copper, iron, manganese, and zinc. Overdoing supplements and multivitamin products can be more harmful than helpful in this regard and, once again, getting these trace elements from food would be a better choice.

There is considerable evidence now that vitamins do not act alone. Hundreds of phytonutrients accompany a vitamin in natural foods and support the absorption and use of the vitamin in the body. So, in the best of all worlds, we will get our vitamins naturally. In the case of vitamin D, we can achieve this with relatively small doses of exposure to the sun, and for the other vitamins from consuming the foods in which they typically occur. Remember, to derive the best level of nutrition, eat unprocessed food with nothing added or taken away. Whenever possible eat beef, fish, poultry, milk products, and eggs from animals that are allowed to eat their own natural diet, rather than an excess of grain that they would not normally consume if they were in the wild. Eat nuts. Incorporate a variety of colors of fresh produce to ensure you take in a variety of antioxidants, vitamins, and other nutrients. And drink organic whole-fat milk.

Clearly, dietary supplements have a role in the fight against Alzheimer's and other such diseases. However, no medication or supplement can undo the ill effects of an unhealthy diet or can take the place of a healthy diet. The primary role of dietary supplements is to supplement the healthy diet as secondary insurance to make sure that certain important nutrients are provided.

It is beyond the scope of this book to attempt to cover all the possible supplements that one might take to prevent or lessen the effects of neurodegenerative diseases. Dozens of supplements purportedly could help. However, one important supplement goes hand in hand with coconut oil and that is the essential omega-3 fatty acid DHA (see pages 81–83).

Consider Alcohol Intake

A number of health gurus encourage people to drink a glass of wine every day, ostensibly to take advantage of a particular substance in the wine called resveratrol. One should consider that the risks may outweigh the benefits in that the alcohol in wine or other alcoholic beverages may in and of itself cause damage to brain cells. In addition, some beers and hard liquors such as Scotch contain nitrosamine compounds, which appear to cause insulin resistance in the brain (De la Monte, 2009).

Another point to consider is that consuming alcohol could greatly increase the confusion and forgetfulness that people with Alzheimer's experience. Steve made a conscious choice to forgo

HOW MUCH OMEGA-3 FATTY ACIDS ARE ENOUGH?

You can obtain all the fatty acids required in the diet by using just coconut oil and omega-3 fatty acids. The body can make all of the fatty acids it needs if these are provided. So, if you decide to use coconut oil as your primary oil, the only other oil you would need is one that contains omega-3 fatty acids. Many people pay no attention to how much omega-3 they are getting. Deficiency in this important fat is rampant in the United States and could at least partly explain the increase in some diseases.

You can get omega-3 fats by eating salmon and other fatty fish, including herring, mackerel, mussels, sardines, swordfish, tilefish, and trout, and by taking liquid or capsules of fish oil, algae oil, or cod liver oil. (Cod liver oil also contains significant amounts of vitamins A, D, and E.) Some good plant sources of omega-3 are ground flaxseed and flax oil, chia seeds and chia oil, camelina oil, walnuts and walnut oil, lingonberries, and purslane. However, because the basic omega-3 fatty acid found in plant sources, alpha-linolenic acid (ALA), may not readily convert to the docosahexaenoic acid (DHA) and eicosapentaenoic acid (EPA) omega-3 fatty acids, marine sources will provide a better guarantee that your brain will get adequate DHA and EPA (Astarita, 2010).

In general, omega-3 fatty acids are metabolized in the body to substances that reduce inflammation, dilate blood vessels, and thin blood, whereas substances derived from metabolism of omega-6 fatty acids have the opposite effects of promoting inflammation and causing blood vessels to constrict and blood to clot. These properties of omega-3 and omega-6 fats are vital to the integrity of the immune system and many other bodily functions and fats should be kept in balance to avoid the problems that could ensue if one fat is routinely consumed in excess over the other. Lipid experts recommend a ratio of omega-6 to omega-3 fats somewhere between 4:1 and 1:1 to avoid problems.

Soybean oil and corn oil contain relatively small amounts of omega-3 fatty acids but much higher amounts of omega-6 fatty acids such that the ratio of omega-6 to omega-3 is very high. These oils could be a source of mysterious inflammation and possibly even high blood pressure for people who regularly consume them as their primary oils and don't get enough omega-3 in the diet to compensate.

DHA makes up 50 percent of a neuron's cell membrane, and low levels of DHA have been associated with Alzheimer's disease as well as many other conditions. DHA is so important that strong consideration should be given to getting this fatty acid directly from a marine source. EPA also plays an important but different role in the cell membrane. For those who object to consuming fish oil, algae oil may be a good alternative. Algae oil is the usual source of omega-3 for products marketed to pregnant women and vegans.

Since each tablespoon of coconut oil contains about 270 mg of omega-6, in order to maintain between a 4:1 and 1:1 ratio of omega-6 to omega-3, one would need to take 70 to 270 mg of omega-3 for each tablespoon of coconut oil consumed in a day. The FDA considers that up to 3,000 mg of marine omega-3 fatty acids are generally recognized as safe (GRAS). A dose of 900 mg of DHA (equivalent to eight standard fish oil capsules) was used a few years ago in a study of people with Alzheimer's disease and mild cognitive impairment, so this dose may be a good level to strive for at the minimum if you are worried about Alzheimer's or other neurodegenerative diseases. You can also get 900 mg of DHA per day from the following alternatives:

- 2 concentrated DHA soft-gel capsules (500 mg DHA per capsule)
- 3 algae oil capsules (320 mg DHA per capsule)
- 8 standard fish oil capsules (120 mg DHA per capsule)
- 9 cod liver oil capsules (100 mg DHA per capsule)
- 2 teaspoons liquid fish oil (500 mg DHA per teaspoon)

> • 7 to 8 ounces baked salmon or other fatty fish (400 mg DHA in
>   3$^1/_2$ ounces)
>
> **CAUTION:** Discuss DHA with the physician first, especially if you are
> taking blood thinners or have other serious health issues.
>
> Source: USDA Food Composition Database, www.nal.usda.gov/
> fnic/foodcomp/search and package labels.

beer, wine, and other alcoholic beverages for that reason, as well as
to prevent further damage to his brain from alcohol.

Consider the Risks of Medications

We all know that many illegal drugs are bad for the brain, but there
is a common misconception that prescription and over-the-counter
drugs must be okay since they have passed muster with the FDA.
Nothing could be further from the truth.

For example, consider acetylcholine. This nervous system neurotransmitter is involved in communication between brain cells and is
diminished in people with Alzheimer's. Anticholinergic drugs,
which include many prescription and nonprescription drugs such
as certain antidepressants, antihistamines, incontinence medications, narcotic pain relievers, and sleep aids, block the attachment
of acetylcholine to its receptors in the brain and may contribute to
symptoms of fogginess, confusion, and memory impairment. This
class of drugs may also counter the effects of Alzheimer's medications, such as donepezil (Aricept) and rivastigmine (Exelon), which
are designed to increase availability of acetylcholine.

Benzodiazepines, corticosteroids, and antipsychotics can cause
side effects (some quite severe) that may be incorrectly attributed to
worsening of the person's dementia. Antipsychotics, for instance,
can affect the brain cells that make dopamine (a chemical that

allows neurons to communicate), resulting in abnormal movements and Parkinson's-type symptoms such as tremor and rigidity in people with Alzheimer's disease, seriously adding to their disabilities. Antipsychotics can also significantly increase blood sugar, which is not a good idea for someone with diabetes, much less diabetes of the brain. Statins (cholesterol-lowering drugs) may cause memory impairment and confusion. These are just a few examples of drugs commonly used in older people and in people with dementia that can have adverse effects. In addition, many drugs and breakdown products of drugs not intended for the brain at all can accumulate in the brain and damage surrounding brain structures directly or possibly by provoking inflammation.

I am not suggesting that everyone should stop all of their medications, but each medication should be strongly considered as to whether it is necessary and if the benefits outweigh the risks. When someone is on multiple medications, careful consideration should be given to whether the drugs might interact with each other. If new problems appear, it is often difficult to know for certain whether they represent worsening of the disease or if they are side effects of the drugs—especially since these side effects may show up weeks to months after starting the medication. Each medication should be reevaluated every few months to determine if it is still necessary or if the dosage can be reduced. In some cases, aggressive or violent behavior may appear at some point and require medication to control the behavior, in which case the benefits of treating may outweigh the risks. As the disease progresses, this behavior may disappear, so at that point the risks may outweigh the benefits and consideration should be given to undertaking a trial off the medication.

For a more extensive discussion of medications that may mimic, worsen, or possibly even cause Alzheimer's disease and the relevant references, see Chapter 15 (2nd edition) of my book *Alzheimer's Disease: What If There Was a Cure?*

3

More About Coconut Oil with Questions and Answers

The coconut palm is called the "tree of life" by people in the Philippines, since every part of the tree has a useful purpose, mainly as food or shelter. Coconuts have been widely used in warmer climates where coconut palms grow, including in parts of Africa, Asia, the Pacific, and other island countries for millennia. Its oil, milk, juice, and meat are staples in the diet of an estimated one-third of the world's population.

Coconuts are nutrient rich. They are a good natural source of iron, phosphorus, zinc, and many other minerals and vitamins. They are also a rich source of protein and fiber, and contain few naturally occurring sugars. Most of the carbohydrate in coconuts is fiber. Coconut oil is made from pressing the meat of coconuts.

In America, in the 1950s, many people cooked with coconut oil and you could buy coconut oil at your local grocery store. People used butter, lard, cottonseed oil, and coconut oil to fry foods in, and it was also used in baking and for making popcorn. Unlike most oils, natural coconut oil is solid at room temperature, does not easily become rancid due to its relatively high amount of saturated fat, and has a shelf life of at least two years. Then, along came Crisco, a partially hydrogenated fat that was heavily marketed to the public. In the hydrogenation process, polyunsaturated vegetable oil is subjected to high heat and pressure, while hydrogen is introduced into the oil. Hydrogen atoms are added to some of the bonds and trans fats are created in the process. The end result is a fat that goes from liquid to solid at room temperature with a much longer shelf life.

From a corporate point of view, when this fat was introduced to the public, coconut oil, with its very long shelf life, was the main competition. With minimal, heavily flawed evidence to support the claim, coconut oil was declared an "artery-clogging" fat and tariffs were placed on it to make it much more expensive, effectively eliminating this rival. The irony is that we now know the newer man-made oils are the true artery-clogging fats that are putting us at greater risk for heart attacks and other deaths from coronary artery (heart) disease, as well as interfering with the metabolism of other fats, including the important and essential omega-3 and omega-6 fatty acids. A diet high in trans fats has been shown in research studies to increase the likelihood of many other health problems, including but not limited to cancer, depression, high blood pressure, infertility, learning disabilities, liver dysfunction, low birth weight, obesity, and, highly relevant to our discussion, Alzheimer's disease and type 2 diabetes. In the fall of 2013 the FDA announced that trans fats no longer have GRAS (generally recognized as safe) status, and that industrially produced trans fats will be phased out and eventually banned from the American diet over the subsequent two years.

Trans fats give a fatty-acid molecule a straighter shape, a higher melting point, and a more rigid structure. The membrane of every cell in the body and the membranes of the organelles within each cell are made up largely of fatty acids. These fatty acids are lined up like tiny magnets side by side and end to end to form what is called a lipid bilayer, a two-layered barrier that repels water and that therefore keeps the watery contents inside the cell from leaking out and the watery fluids outside the cell from getting in. Putting trans fats into a cell membrane is like trying to put a square peg into a round hole. The human body is not programmed through evolution to use these altered fats and, as a result, the trans fats do not line up normally with the other molecules in the lipid bilayer (see Figure 3.1). This misalignment decreases the fluidity of the cell and the functioning of the cell membrane, and may even shorten the lifespan of the cell.

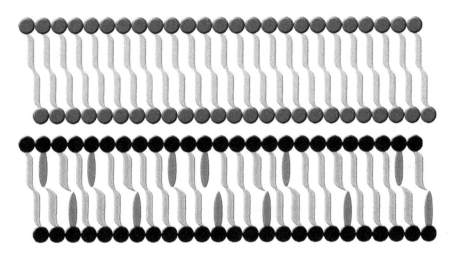

FIGURE 3.1. (Top diagram) Lipid bilayer without trans fats is more fluid and flexible. (Bottom diagram) Lipid bilayer with trans fats is more rigid.

When partially hydrogenated fats came on the market, many physicians and researchers expressed concerns about these manufactured fats, questioning whether they were truly safe, but their voices were not heard for many years. The use of trans fats is already banned in some parts of the world. Until the recently announced phase-out, the powers that be in the United States had taken the position that providing trans fat contents on package labels was adequate protection for consumers. However, until the phase-out is complete, it should be duly noted that if the trans fat content of a food is less than 0.5 grams per serving, the manufacturer is permitted to list the trans fat content as "0." Thus, if the serving size is adjusted accordingly to ensure the trans fat content is less than 0.5 grams, the consumer could well be getting significant trans fats in the product and not know it. Labeling changes are also coming down the pike requiring that more realistic serving sizes be stated on food labels. The best way to avoid trans fats is to look at the list of ingredients and avoid products that contain the words "hydrogenated" or "partially hydrogenated."

Physicians who tell their patients to avoid coconut oil rarely suggest that they should also avoid the trans fats in partially hydrogenated vegetable oils. They may not even be aware of the true artery-clogging potential of these manufactured fats that are used in very many kitchens, convenience foods, and fast-food restaurants. Many physicians regularly consume partially hydrogenated fats themselves without batting an eye. I know because I used to be one of them!

MISCONCEPTIONS ABOUT COCONUT OIL, SATURATED FAT, AND CHOLESTEROL

The major objections to using coconut oil center on long-held beliefs that coconut oil is a saturated fat that raises cholesterol levels, and that saturated fat and high cholesterol levels cause heart disease. The "lipid hypothesis" of heart disease, which was the basis for the decades-long public policy encouraging a low-fat diet, was based on highly flawed research that was unsuccessfully challenged by other researchers at the time. If fat is decreased in the diet, carbohydrates will naturally fill the gap in the diet. We have already learned the results of this vast experiment, which has led to pandemics of obesity, diabetes, dementia, and other serious conditions. Here is the latest basic information on these fats.

Saturated Fat

There is a misconception that all saturated fats, particularly those found in meat and dairy products, are bad and should be avoided in the diet at all costs. But saturated fats are made naturally by our bodies and are essential to our health. For instance, palmitic acid, one of the most common long-chain saturated fats, is a major fatty acid in normal lung surfactant, a substance made inside each of the alveoli (air sacs) in the lungs that keeps the alveoli open. Without surfactant, the lungs would collapse and we would die in short order. This happens in the real world when people die from smoke inhalation, which inactivates surfactant, and when very premature newborns die from the inability of the lungs to make enough surfactant. Certain saturated fats are important to white blood cell function, a major component of our response to infection; they also help stabilize many different proteins, including those in the immune system, and fight tumors. Certain other saturated fatty acids are important to signaling of hormones. In addition, long-chain saturated fatty acids are found in neurons and in myelin (the protective sheath around the nerves), and very-long-chain saturated fatty acids are important components of cell membranes, especially in the brain.

Interestingly, in humans, the fat beneath the skin (subcutaneous fat) is roughly 27 percent saturated, 50 percent monounsaturated, and 23 percent polyunsaturated—give or take a few percent in either direction depending largely on what we eat (Ren, 2008). The amount of fat we carry in our bodies has less to do with how much saturated or unsaturated fat we eat, and more to do with how many calories we eat, be they in the form of fat, protein, or carbohydrates. When the intake of calories is too high in relation to how much energy is expended, the liver converts glucose and protein, as well as fatty acids, into fat in the form of triglycerides, which are released into the bloodstream and then stored in fat tissue. This is a simplified explanation for a very complex process. When a person's serum triglyceride levels are chronically elevated, it usually has more to do with consuming too many calories and too much sugar than too much fat.

Many conflicting studies have attempted to clarify the relationship between saturated fat and heart disease. A report published in 2014 analyzed data for nearly 660,000 participants in seventy-six studies of fatty acids and heart disease, of which twenty-seven were randomized controlled trials, and found no clear evidence that supports the current recommendations that encourage high consumption of polyunsaturated fats and low consumption of total saturated fats. The researchers found no connection between total saturated fat intake and coronary disease. They did, however, find a greater risk of heart disease with trans fatty acid consumption. They also point out that elevated saturated fat levels in the blood correlate much more strongly with increased consumption of carbohydrates and alcohol, and only very weakly with saturated fat consumption, since the body will increase its own production of certain saturated fats in response to sugar and alcohol intake (Chowdhury, 2014).

Cholesterol

Cholesterol is not actually a fat but a steroid of fat. All cholesterol is made from the basic energy molecule acetyl-CoA, and most of it by far is made in the body rather than consumed in the diet. We tend to produce a certain amount of cholesterol over the course of a day, and when we do not eat enough, our liver will compensate by making more; likewise, if we eat more cholesterol than we need, our liver will make less. This means that reducing cholesterol intake does not affect our total cholesterol level much. The major dietary sources of cholesterol are found in foods of animal origins such as cheese, egg yolks, beef, pork, poultry, and shrimp.

The issue of whether natural non-oxidized cholesterol is involved in heart disease is in question, given that half of people who have heart attacks have cholesterol levels in the "normal" range. There are many conflicting studies about whether higher cholesterol levels may contribute to the development of dementia or actually protect against it (Seneff, 2011). It has been found in people with Alzheimer's that their cerebrospinal fluid (which bathes the brain and spinal cord) is depleted of lipoproteins, cholesterol, triglycerides, and fatty acids compared to the fluid in people without Alzheimer's. In fact, the fatty acid levels in the spinal fluid are depleted by a factor of six compared to the levels in people without Alzheimer's disease (Mulder, 1998).

When cholesterol is involved in hardening of the arteries, heart attacks, and strokes, it is likely that the oxidized form of cholesterol, called oxycholesterol, is a major culprit, along with small, dense LDL cholesterol particles (abbreviated sdLDL) that are more susceptible to oxidation (Toft-Petersen, 2011). While statins do decrease total LDL cholesterol, they do not decrease the amount of harmful sdLDL in the blood and, in fact, they increase the overall percent of sdLDL in the blood relative to the total LDL (Choi, 2010). Foods known to increase levels of sdLDL are sugar and trans fats. Also, higher levels of sdLDL are more common in diabetics (Mauger, 2003; Siri, 2005).

Information about the role of oxycholesterol in heart disease was presented at the 2009 meeting of the American Chemical Society by Zhen-Yu Chen, Ph.D., who learned in his studies at the Chinese University of Hong Kong that people who consume oxycholesterol tend to have greater depositions of this type of cholesterol in the lining of their arteries, as well as larger deposits or plaques, which increase their risk for heart attacks and strokes. Oxycholesterol makes the arteries less flexible and therefore less able to expand as a larger volume of blood attempts to move through them.

Cholesterol becomes oxidized when exposed to oxygen and to high heat as in the grilling of meats. It is also created intentionally when partially hydrogenated fats with trans fats are produced, and so is found in many fast foods and processed foods. When butter is clarified and subjected to high heat, as in the making of ghee, oxycholesterol is formed. Powdered milk and eggs, also found in many processed foods, but rarely labeled as such, may contain substantial oxycholesterol. More recently, high blood pressure and inflammation in blood vessel walls have been implicated as well in the development of heart attacks and strokes, which suggests that there could very well be a connection between oxidized cholesterol in the linings of arteries walls and these other problems.

The cholesterol issue, in general, focuses on levels that are considered to be too high. But low cholesterol levels also appear to play a role in disease. Extremely low cholesterol levels are associated with a higher risk of death from cancer, for example, and are associated with higher mortality in general at a given age (Schatz, 2001).

As with saturated fat, there are serious misconceptions that all cholesterol is bad. Cholesterol is so vital, in fact, that it is contained and made in every cell in the body, and performs a long list of beneficial functions. The body uses cholesterol to produce adrenal and sex hormones, to aid in the manufacture of bile acids needed for the digestion of fats, to help keep the skin healthy, and to provide a source of vitamin D, a necessity for calcium absorption. Cholesterol is required in infancy for normal brain development (large amounts of cholesterol are present in human breast milk). It makes up from 30 to 40 percent of the cell membrane, which helps create the cell's shape and protects it from being bent or deformed. It is a critical component of some cell receptors, which bind to specific chemicals to allow transport of certain substances into the cell, and it is a major component of the protective coating around the myelin sheaths of the nerves in the brain and central nervous system. Communication between nerves and brain cells at the synapses (junctions) cannot take place without the presence of cholesterol. Cholesterol also protects cells from free-radical attack, therefore acting as an antioxidant.

We need a certain amount of cholesterol every day to perform these many essential functions. According to expert fat researcher

Mary Enig, the total body cholesterol for the average 150-pound man is equal to 145,000 milligrams (mg), or about one-third of a pound. From 10,000 to 14,000 mg of this cholesterol is circulating in the bloodstream. What we don't eat is otherwise produced in large part by the liver and the intestines, and can be produced inside every properly functioning cell. As mentioned previously, if we take in too much cholesterol, the liver will make less; if we do not take in enough cholesterol in food, the liver will make more. This is one reason why reducing dietary intake of cholesterol has relatively little, if any, impact on lowering total cholesterol levels. The liver is reported to make as much as 5 grams (5,000 mg) of cholesterol a day; therefore, if a person consumes the currently recommended 300 mg of cholesterol a day, of which only half is absorbed by the intestines, the small amount eaten will have little effect on the total cholesterol level.

If the total cholesterol level increases at all when consuming coconut oil, the "good" HDL cholesterol tends to increase more than the "bad" LDL fraction. HDL and LDL are actually the carriers of cholesterol rather than cholesterol itself, and they carry many other important substances as well.

A word is in order here regarding statins and whether these cholesterol-lowering drugs are harmful or beneficial to people who have dementia or are at risk for dementia. There is a high rate of adverse effects with statin use, more than 40 percent, according to University of California–San Diego researcher Beatrice Golomb, M.D. (Golomb, 2005 and 2008; Evans 2009). The FDA requires statins to carry information on their labels stating that memory loss and confusion may occur and that these drugs carry an increased risk of raised blood sugar levels and development of type 2 diabetes, which we are trying to avoid. Statins are too often prescribed to treat a cholesterol number without much regard to the other risk factors that may or may not predispose the patient to heart disease. Adverse effects such as muscle aches and fatigue are too often dismissed by physicians. Since cholesterol-lowering drugs may play an important role in preventing heart attacks in some people who are at risk, any changes in use of this medication should be discussed with the patient's physician.

For a more extensive discussion of the issues revolving around cholesterol and saturated fat that often come up in relation to coconut oil, see Chapter 21 of my previous book, *Alzheimer's Disease: What If There Was a Cure? The Story of Ketones.*

QUESTIONS AND ANSWERS ABOUT COCONUT OIL

Until commercial ketone-containing foods and drinks are available to us, the next best strategy we can undertake is to incorporate medium-chain triglycerides into our diet. Medium-chain fatty acids are taken up directly from the intestines to the liver, where they are partially converted to ketones. These ketones are then taken up quickly by cells that can use them, including those in the brain, and also serve as an alternative fuel for cells that are unable to use glucose effectively. In addition, medium-chain triglycerides can be used directly as fuel by mitochondria, the tiny organelles inside of cells that generate adenosine triphosphate (ATP), an energy molecule.

There are several ways to incorporate medium-chain triglycerides into the diet: with coconut or palm kernel oil, with medium-chain triglyceride (MCT) oil, and with foods and products rich in these medium-chain fatty acids. This chapter focuses mainly on answering frequently asked questions about coconut oil and coconut oil in foods. The following chapter will answer questions concerning MCT oil and products that contain MCT oil.

What Is the Nutrient Content of Coconut Oil?

Coconut oil has 117 to 120 calories per tablespoon, about the same as other oils. It contains 57 to 60 percent medium-chain triglycerides, which are absorbed directly from the intestines without the need for digestive enzymes. This portion of the coconut oil is not stored as fat. Coconut oil is about 86 percent saturated fat, however, about 70 percent of these saturated fats are the special medium-chain fats that are metabolized differently than the longer-chain saturated fats. One important advantage of a saturated fat isthat there is nowhere on the molecule for free radicals or oxidants to attach. About 6 percent of coconut oil is monounsaturated fat and 2 percent omega-6 polyunsaturated fat. There are no omega-3 fatty acids in coconut oil, so this important essential fat must come from elsewhere—ideally, from a marine source that provides the type of omega-3 needed by cells of the brain and other organs to function normally. In many countries where coconut oil is prevalent in the diet, fish is an important staple as well. When combined, they provide a full complement of fatty acids.

Contrary to popular belief, there is no cholesterol in coconut oil. In fact, the oil contains small amounts of phytosterols, plant compounds that are somewhat similar to cholesterol in structure but that are actually used in certain statins for lowering cholesterol.

Coconut oil contains no trans fat as long as it is not hydrogenated or partially hydrogenated.

Lauric acid is a medium-chain triglyceride that makes up almost half of coconut oil and is a saturated fat. Scientific studies show that lauric acid has antimicrobial properties, which may inhibit growth of certain bacteria, fungi, viruses, and protozoa. It is one of the components of human breast milk that prevents infection in a newborn. Coconut oil and/or palm kernel oil, which have a similar composition of fats, are added to nearly every infant formula to try to duplicate the important fatty acids, such as lauric acid, found in human breast milk. It is remarkable that coconut oil is considered so safe, and even important, for the human newborn and yet is considered by many to be dangerous for the adult human. The inconsistency is mind-boggling.

Because coconut oil contains a small amount of omega-6 fatty acids and no omega-3 fatty acid, omega-3 must be taken in addition to coconut oil either in food or as a supplement.

Should We Bother Trying This Approach If My Loved One with Alzheimer's Has the ApoE4 Gene?

Yes! In a pilot study of AC-1202 (now called Axona, the prescription powdered form of MCT oil from Accera), involving twenty people with memory impairment, the researchers learned that nearly half improved after a single dose of the oil compared to when they received a placebo on another occasion (Reger, 2004). A larger study of 152 people taking AC-1202 over three months had similar results (Costantini, 2008). In both studies, this effect appeared to occur primarily in people who did not carry the apolipoprotein E4 (ApoE4) gene that carries a higher risk of Alzheimer's; however, some individuals with ApoE4 did have improvement in their cognitive test scores. In addition, my husband, Steve, has the ApoE4 gene and responded dramatically to medium-chain triglycerides. These were relatively small studies and larger studies of MCT oil are currently underway to look at whether more frequent dosing and larger amounts might be even more effective in both people who carry the ApoE4 gene and those who do not.

How Much Coconut Oil Should I Take?

If you take too much coconut oil too fast, you may experience indigestion, cramping, or diarrhea. To avoid these symptoms, take coconut oil with food and start with one-half to one teaspoon per meal, increasing slowly as tolerated over a week or longer. If diarrhea develops, drop back to the previous level and stay at that level for at least a few days before trying to increase the amount again. (See Chapter 4 for more ideas on reducing the problem of diarrhea.)

For most people, the goal is to increase gradually to three to six tablespoons a day, depending on the size of the person, spread over two to four meals. Not everyone will be able to tolerate this much oil and some may be able to tolerate as much as nine to twelve tablespoons per day. Some people who have remained stable with their disease process for two to four years are taking these larger amounts of coconut oil.

In the intriguing book *Coconut Oil Secrets Exposed* (2013), authors Charles Chou and Debbie Ng recount the experiences of a Taiwanese folk doctor in Sumatra who had her patients drink one or two cups of coconut oil per day. She effectively "cured" many, including women with breast cancer; an individual with kidney failure; a diabetic with a severely rotting leg; and a person who was comatose for ten years, woke up, and began to speak and eventually walk again. At first consideration, such claims might seem impossible and could easily be dismissed. However, someone who is receiving sixteen tablespoons (one cup) or more of coconut oil on a daily basis would effectively be on the equivalent of a classic low-carb, high-fat ketogenic diet. There is now growing evidence supporting the use of the ketogenic diet to treat cancer (Poff, 2014), as well as a study in which diabetic kidney disease was completely reversed in mice on a ketogenic diet (Poplawski, 2011). And I have personally received case reports of two people who came out of a coma after receiving MCT oil, and another who recovered significantly from a severe lack of oxygen, after his progress had stalled, when he began consuming coconut oil. Given the dramatic response that my husband had to consuming coconut oil, I have to consider that such coconut oil- and ketone-related "cures" are within the realm of possibility.

A man with ALS (also known as Lou Gehrig's disease) has had success in bringing about improvement, and then stabilization, in his condition for more than four years from taking nine tablespoons of coconut oil a day and also by massaging the oil over his muscles.

His response is quite remarkable considering that this disease is relentless in its progression and most people die within three to five years of diagnosis. He is now helping many others with ALS learn how to use this intervention, and evaluate and document their progress. (You can read his story in Chapter 10.) He and I agree that there are many people who initially embrace this dietary commitment but eventually slack off, even in the face of improvement, and lose the edge they have on the disease. He recently told me that it took several months of consuming large amounts of coconut oil to notice that he had stabilized, and more months until he saw improvement. The improvements are a good sign that ketones are doing their job, but the underlying disease process is still present in the body. To get the maximum benefit from this strategy, developing a plan for increasing the daily intake of coconut oil, MCT oil, or a combination of the two, and then sticking with it indefinitely are key. For those who respond, this will be a lifetime dietary change.

Two men with Parkinson's disease have reported similar success while taking nine or more tablespoons per day of coconut oil. For each, the improvements were gradual but ultimately profound.

Mixing MCT oil and coconut oil could provide higher levels, and a steady level, of ketones and might be more effective for some people than coconut oil alone—although it is hard to argue with the success that the people mentioned above have achieved with coconut oil alone. One formula is to mix 16 ounces of MCT oil plus 12 ounces of coconut oil in a quart glass jar and increase slowly as tolerated, starting with one teaspoon. This mixture will stay liquid at room temperature. For those who are still concerned about consuming saturated fats, a four-to-three ratio of MCT oil to coconut oil will keep the level of long-chain saturated fats in this mixture at roughly 10 percent of the total fat content. (The complete recipe for making MCT and Coconut Oil 4:3 Mixture is found in Chapter 5.) Over one year's time, Steve increased his daily intake of this coconut and MCT oil mixture to eleven tablespoons, divided into three tablespoons with each meal and two tablespoons with an evening snack before bedtime. This represents nearly half the calories in his diet. The goal is to keep ketones available to his brain round the clock.

How Can Coconut Oil Be Used in the Diet?

Coconut oil can be substituted for any solid or liquid oil, lard, butter, or margarine in baking or stove-top cooking, and it can be mixed directly into foods that are already prepared. Although some people take it straight with a spoon, many people may find it difficult to swallow this way and more pleasant to take with food. Try using coconut oil instead of butter on whole-grain varieties of toast, English muffins, bagels, grits, corn on the cob, potatoes, sweet potatoes, rice, vegetables, and noodles. If you decide to adopt a lower-carbohydrate diet along with this coconut oil strategy, limit the foods in this list to one or two small servings a day, with the exception of non-starchy vegetables. If you decide to eliminate gluten as well, this list of foods will be further reduced. The coconut oil works best when added to vegetables that are still warm after cooking or that are sautéed with coconut oil.

Remember, when stir-frying or sautéing on the stove, coconut oil smokes if heated to more than 350°F (175°C), or above medium heat. You can avoid this by adding a little olive, canola, or peanut oil to the pan beforehand.

Coconut oil can be used at any temperature in the oven when it is mixed into the ingredients. Mix coconut oil into your favorite soup, chili, or sauce. It can also be basted on foods such as fish as long as the oven temperature is 350°F or below.

Coconut oil tends to become hard when exposed to cold foods. For instance, if used as a salad dressing, the oil will turn into hard little chunks if the vegetables in the salad come straight from the refrigerator. Some people actually like this effect and call them "crunchies"; if not, try adding equal amounts of coconut oil to another favorite salad dressing that has been warmed slightly. Also, the MCT and Coconut Oil 4:3 Mixture (mentioned earlier) tends to stay liquid and works well in this situation; it also works well in smoothies, yogurt, or kefir.

For those who cannot handle coconut oil, unsweetened grated or flaked coconut, coconut milk, and fresh coconut may be good substitutes, as they are digested much more slowly. Ideas for incorporating these foods into the diet are discussed later in the chapter.

Caregivers have found very creative ways to get coconut oil into the diet of their loved ones, particularly those with a sweet tooth who are resistant to taking the oil with other foods. Two favorite recipes found in Chapter 5 are Coconut Macaroons and Coconut Fudge. Also, check the Resources section for cookbooks containing many more great ideas and recipes.

What Kind of Coconut Oil Should I Use?

Be sure to examine the product label on the jar or container. Look for coconut oils that are non-hydrogenated with no trans fat. Avoid coconut oils that are partially hydrogenated or super-heated because these processes change the chemical structure of the fats. In the United States, food manufacturers are required to state on the label whether their product contains hydrogenated or partially hydrogenated oils and trans fats. One caution, as noted earlier, is that labels may list no trans fats if a serving contains less than 0.5 grams. This can be deceptive, since the serving size is often adjusted accordingly.

Two basic types of coconut oil are on the market: unrefined and refined. The label for unrefined coconut oil normally reads "virgin" or "extra-virgin," may read "raw," and most often also reads "organic." These unrefined oils are generally pressed from freshly harvested coconuts and are rarely exposed to high levels of heat. As a result, they are more flavorful and nutritious than refined coconut oils; they also tend to be more expensive, largely because the nature of the equipment and the process used in removing the oils from the meat are more costly to the manufacturer. There are quality differences with more than six different ways of making virgin coconut oil. Generally, some type of mechanical process, such as a press or a centrifuge, is used rather than chemicals to separate the oil from the coconut meat. One example is a process called direct micro-expelling (DME), which was developed by Dan Etherington, an Australian who pioneered virgin coconut oil production in the South Pacific. DME is a cold (low-heat) process of pressing the oil from the fresh meat within one hour of opening the coconut.

Refined coconut oil is made from copra (dried coconut flesh), which, in the drying process and transit time to the oil mills, often picks up mold and off-flavors, and thus needs to be refined to be palatable. The label usually reads "regular," "all natural," or "RBD" (refined, bleached, and deodorized). The dried coconut is soaked in bleach and solvents are used to leach out the oils, which are subjected to high temperatures to further purify and liquefy the oils. Refined coconut oils have virtually no coconut taste or aroma.

Coconut oil can be found at natural food stores, most Asian markets, some traditional grocery stores, as well as large department stores with grocery sections. More recently, large 54-ounce containers of organic cold-pressed virgin coconut oil can be purchased at buyers' clubs such as Sam's Club and Costco for less than $16. You can also use the Internet to find other quality brands of coconut oil and at a wide range of prices not available at your local retailer. Check the Resources section for a listing of websites offering coconut oil and coconut oil products.

What About Using Coconut Oil Capsules?

Using coconut oil capsules is not an efficient way to get the oil. The capsules are relatively expensive and nearly all contain only 1 gram

(1,000 mg) of oil per capsule, whereas there are 14 grams (14,000 mg) in one tablespoon of oil. Some products state there are 4 grams (4,000 mg) per serving; however, the serving size is four capsules. It would require taking about fourteen capsules to equal one tablespoon of coconut oil and, as such, may not be practical and could be expensive to use capsules. On the other hand, for people who will not use the oil in liquid form and have no problem with swallowing capsules, this may offer an alternative. (See the Resources section.)

Why Does Coconut Oil Look Cloudy?

Coconut oil is a clear or slightly yellow liquid above 76°F but becomes solid at 76°F and below. If the temperature of your house is kept right around 76°F, the oil may even become partly liquid oil with solid clouds floating in it. If your home is generally kept at 75°F or below, the oil will tend to be white or slightly yellow, and soft to semi-solid.

What Other Coconut Products Contain Coconut Oil?

Coconut milk is a combination of the oil and the water from the coconut. Most of the calories are from the oil. Look for brands with 10 to 13 grams of fat in 2 ounces. Coconut milk also contains some protein and a small amount of carbohydrate, which gives it a slightly sweet taste. Coconut milk can generally be found in natural foods stores, Asian markets, and the Asian and/or Hispanic sections of traditional grocery stores. Look at the fat content closely on the label, and be aware that some less-expensive brands are considerably diluted with water. There are also brands of coconut milk available in one-half gallon containers (found in the cold-milk section of stores and on the shelf) that are often very dilute with water and somewhat bland. These contain about 45 to 80 calories per 8-ounce serving and would require consuming 12 to 20 ounces to equal just one tablespoon of coconut oil. You can dilute condensed coconut milk yourself with water, or even better, with coconut water, which is loaded with vitamins and other nutrients, and adds flavor to the mixture. Coconut milk powder and organic coconut milk are also available. Some coconut milks are labeled "light" or "lite." Much of the oil has been removed, and using these lower-fat products defeats our purpose of including coconut oil in the diet. Coconut milk blends very well into smoothies and is a tasty substitute for cow's milk on hot or cold cereal or right out of the glass. Coconut milk can be substituted for some or all the milk in many recipes. See the Coconut Milk recipes in Chapter 5 for suggested dilutions of canned coconut milk.

The term coconut butter is sometimes used to refer to coconut oil in its solid state (at 75°F/24°C or below) or it may refer to coconut manna or creamed coconut (pureed coconut meat), which is whole coconut blended into a paste that is fairly solid at room temperature.

Some wonderful ice creams are now available in a variety of flavors made with coconut milk as the first ingredient. Coconut-milk ice creams are available at Asian markets, many natural food stores, and some traditional grocery stores. There are even some ice cream products labeled "gluten-free." Coconut ice cream may be one way to encourage coconut oil intake for someone with a sweet tooth or for an otherwise uncooperative loved one.

Coconut cream is mostly coconut milk, often has added sugar, and comes in liquid and powdered forms.

Flaked, chipped, or grated coconut can be purchased unsweetened or sweetened and is a very good source of coconut oil and fiber. Grated coconut has about 14 grams of oil and 3 grams of fiber in one-fourth cup; in fact, about 70 percent of its carbohydrate content is fiber. The oil in grated coconut can help with absorption of certain vitamins and other nutrients as well. Flaked, chipped, or grated coconut can be bought in bulk, often for about

$3 per pound, at many natural food stores, or packaged in natural food sections of grocery stores. It can be added to cold or hot cereals, smoothies, soup, and ricotta or cottage cheese, and used as a topper for ice cream. Flaked coconut is often found in trail mix, and some people snack on unsweetened flaked coconut. Store-bought or homemade macaroons, made with grated coconut, are a delicious source of coconut oil. (See Chapter 5 for a recipe.)

Frozen or canned coconut meat often has a lot of added sugar and not much oil per serving. Coconut meat can also be found in jars as coconut balls and "coconut sport," which are large strands of coconut. These products are especially nice for adding to fruit salads.

A fresh coconut can be cut up into pieces and eaten raw. A two-inch square piece has about 160 calories with 15 grams of oil (equivalent to about one tablespoon oil) and 4 grams of fiber. Removing the meat from the coconut can be quite a challenge, however. In Bruce Fife's *The Coconut Lover's Cookbook* (2008), he suggests heating the whole coconut in an oven for twenty min-

---

SOME COCONUT OIL EQUIVALENTS

The following coconut foods and supplements contain the equivalent of 1 tablespoon of coconut oil:

- Coconut butter: usually 1 tablespoon
- Coconut chips: about $1/4$ to $1/3$ cup
- Coconut flaked or grated, unsweetened: about $1/4$ to $1/3$ cup
- Coconut manna: $1 1/2$ tablespoons
- Coconut meat: 2-by-2-by-$1/2$-inch piece
- Coconut milk (undiluted): $4 1/2$ tablespoons
- Coconut milk powder: 3 tablespoons
- Coconut oil capsules (1 gram): 14 capsules

utes at 400°F after poking two holes in the eyes of the coconut and draining the coconut water. After the coconut cools down, it can be opened with a hammer or whatever tool you can think of. To avoid shattering anything important, take the coconut outside and crack it open on newspapers. The meat can usually be pried from the shell with a blunt knife or one of the special tools that may be available at Asian stores to scrape the coconut out of the shell. This is quite a process and can be time consuming, but some consider it well worth it. Pieces of coconut meat can be saved for a week or longer in the freezer.

Coconut water does not usually contain coconut oil but does contain many other nutrients, and has other health benefits. Its electrolyte composition is similar to human plasma and is useful to prevent or treat dehydration. It is an excellent source of potassium with 360 mg in an 8-ounce serving. Coconut water has been used as intravenous fluid in Asia and was even used by our American troops in World War II when supplies of standard intravenous fluids were low. Coconut water is coming into its own now as a sports drink (plain and flavored) and is readily available in mainstream grocery stores.

MCT oil is part of the coconut oil and can also be purchased in some natural food stores or on the Internet. Using MCT oil instead of coconut oil may be useful for people who are on the go and do not have much time to cook with coconut oil. Now, even mainstream grocery stores and pharmacies are carrying "coconut cooking oil," a product in which some of the longer-chain fats have been removed from the oil so that it is more concentrated in medium-chain triglycerides.

How Should Coconut Products Be Stored?

Coconut oil is extremely stable with a shelf life of at least two years when stored at room temperature. The container should have an expiration date on it. In the refrigerator, coconut oil becomes quite hard, so you may need a chisel to get it out of the jar! If you wish to keep it in the refrigerator, you can measure out one or two table-spoons into each section of a plastic ice cube tray. The coconut oil pops easily out of the tray. Refrigeration is not necessary, but some people may be more comfortable storing it this way.

Coconut milk is mostly coconut oil and can be substituted for the oil in many ways. Coconut milk must be refrigerated after open-ing, and should be used within a few days or tossed out.

Grated or flaked coconut can be stored at room temperature but may last longer if stored in a refrigerator.

A freshly cut coconut can be stored in the refrigerator for a few days or in the freezer for a couple of weeks.

What Other Foods Contain Medium-Chain Triglycerides?

Some other foods contain medium-chain triglycerides that are worth mentioning, including full-fat cow's milk, goat's milk, sheep's milk and cheeses, as well as other dairy products made from these animals. Table 3.1 (page 107) shows the content (in grams per serv-ing) of the medium-chain fatty acids contained in these and other foods. In general, the amounts are considerably less than in coconut oil. However, using these foods may contribute to the overall pro-duction of ketones. In other parts of the world, certain oils may be more available than in the United States, such as babassu oil, which contains 7.7 grams per tablespoon (15 ml), and ucuhuba butter with 1.8 grams per tablespoon.

Are There Commercial Products That Contain a Mixture of Coconut and MCT Oils?

In its natural state at room temperature, coconut oil is usually solid and can be challenging to measure and mix with other foods. Two

TABLE 3.1. FOODS WITH MEDIUM-CHAIN TRIGLYCERIDES

FATS AND OILS	GRAMS PER 0.5 OUNCE (APPROXIMATELY 3 TSP/15 ML)
Coconut oil	8.3
Babassu oil	7.7
Palm kernel oil	7.5
Goat butter	2.4
Ucuhuba butter	1.8
Cow butter	1.6
Nutmeg butter	0.4
Shea nut butter	0.24
Lard	0.04

CREAM AND CHEESE	GRAMS PER OUNCE (APPROXIMATELY 6 TSP/30 ML)
Goat cheese	2.0
Feta cheese	1.4
Cream (heavy)	1.3
Cream cheese	1.0
American cheese	0.85
Mozzarella	0.78

MILKS AND COTTAGE CHEESE	GRAMS PER 8 OUNCES (APPROXIMATELY 1 CUP/240 ML)
Goat milk	1.7
Infant formula	1.0
Cow milk (full-fat)	0.9
Human breast milk	0.78
Cottage cheese	0.78

NOTE: The following commonly eaten fats and oils contain no short- and medium-chain fatty acids: canola, cod liver, corn, fish, flaxseed, olive, peanut, safflower, soybean and sunflower oils, as well as margarine.

SOURCE: USDA National Nutrient Database for Standard Reference, Release 23. Agricultural Research Service (www.ars.usda.gov/nutrientdata), 2010.

new products now on the market make the process of incorporating coconut oil into the diet considerably easier: One product is Fuel for Thought from Cognate Nutritionals. This creamy mixture of coconut, highly enriched with MCT oil, and natural fruit flavors is packaged in two-serving bottles that can be taken as is or added to other foods or liquids. The formulation contains no preservatives or other additives and can be kept at room temperature on the day it is opened. Each serving has more than double the amount of ketone-producing medium-chain triglycerides as three tablespoons of coconut oil. This product is comprised exclusively of ingredients classified by the FDA and the USDA as GRAS. The availability of Fuel for Thought is particularly useful to anyone needing assistance, as well as those who want an easy, convenient way to add coconut oil and MCT oil to the diet. The small bottles also make this product very useful for travel and also for eating out.

A second product, developed by Alpha Health Products in Canada, called MCT Coconut Gourmet Salad Oil, combines MCT oil with DME virgin coconut oil in the four-to-three ratio that Steve and I have used. An unrefined omega-3-rich vegetable oil is also added and gives a pleasant nutty taste. This oil mixture is liquid and stable at room temperature due to its high-MCT content and will easily combine with lemon or vinegar to make salad dressing. (See Chapter 5 for additional salad dressing recipes.)

Can Someone Who Is in Assisted Living Take Coconut Oil?

If your loved one is in assisted living, the doctor may be willing to prescribe coconut oil to be given at each meal and can order the oils to be increased gradually as tolerated. A number of people have reported success in this regard. Fuel for Thought (discussed above) is packaged in two-serving bottles and is convenient for this situation. The physician can be asked to write an order so that a serving of a product such as Fuel for Thought can be given to your loved one at mealtimes. I know of one assisted living facility in which the cook was preparing some foods with coconut oil. She said the residents with Alzheimer's disease seemed more talkative and to have more energy. Hopefully, over time, the directors of these facilities will consider allowing staff to cook with coconut oil. If no such options are possible, another alternative is to ask the your loved one's physician for a prescription for Axona, a powdered form of MCT oil, manufactured by Accera (more on this product in Chapter 4).

What About Someone with Liver Disease Using Coconut Oil?

This dietary intervention may not be appropriate for someone with severe liver disease. A healthy liver is required to convert medium-chain triglycerides to ketones. Partially hydrogenated oils, including partially hydrogenated coconut oil, can result in a fatty liver. Therefore, it is important to always use non-hydrogenated coconut oil or any other oil, for that matter.

Do I Need to Worry About Gaining Weight from the Extra Fat in the Diet?

No and yes! Some studies show that substitution of coconut oil for other fats in the diet can actually result in weight loss of ten to twelve pounds over the course of a year, because the medium-chain triglycerides are converted directly to energy and not stored as fat. However, if coconut oil is simply added to the diet and nothing subtracted, you can expect to gain weight. In general, if you consume more calories than you burn in the course of a day, the net result will be weight gain—although this process is more complicated than just described. The best way to avoid gaining weight is to substitute coconut oil for most other fats and oils in the diet, and if that isn't enough, eliminate or cut back on portion sizes of carbohydrates, such as breads, rice, potatoes, cereals, and other grains.

In general, it is a good idea to use full-fat dairy products, but if weight gain is a problem, you can compensate for some of the new fat in the diet by changing to lower-fat milk, cheese, cottage cheese, and yogurt products, as well as to low-fat or fat-free salad dressings, to which you can add coconut or MCT oil. By the same token, if you decide to go with low-fat dairy, be aware that you may not absorb as much calcium and vitamin D through the intestines, when compared with full-fat dairy. Also, some people overestimate portions substantially by dipping into the coconut oil jar with a kitchen tablespoon. You can avoid this problem by using a measuring spoon and removing the excess by leveling it off with a knife. Proper measuring can make a big difference in the number of calories consumed. Tiny glass measuring cups are available at grocery stores with markings for teaspoons, tablespoons, and milliliters. These little measuring cups are especially useful for combining salad dressing with coconut oil and for measuring out the liquid MCT and Coconut Oil 4:3 Mixture discussed elsewhere.

A plan for limiting carbohydrate intake is discussed in more detail in Chapter 2.

Can Coconut Oil Be Given to Children?

Yes! Human breast milk includes 10 to 17 percent of its fat as medium-chain triglycerides. To give you an idea of just how important medium-chain fatty acids are to humans, a ten-pound breast-feeding baby gets about 3.12 grams of medium-chain triglycerides per quart of breast milk. Extrapolated to a 150-pound adult, that would be the equivalent of 47 grams of medium-chain triglycerides and would require eating five and a half tablespoons of coconut oil.

To try to duplicate what is in human breast milk, every infant formula manufactured in the United States contains MCT oil as well as coconut and/or palm kernel oil. The only exceptions I am aware of for adding coconut oil or MCT oil to the diet are in children and adults with liver failure, an allergy to coconut, and certain rare enzyme deficiencies (for a list of conditions that result in defective lipid metabolism, see Appendix 1). When children are weaned from the breast and from infant formulas, the usual next step in the United States is to transition to cow's milk. In recent years, there has been a push to encourage feeding even small children low-fat or fat-free milk and milk products, which would eliminate every potential source of medium-chain triglycerides from the diet of the average child.

I have had many parents of children with autism and Down syndrome (also called trisomy 21) ask about using coconut oil. Several parents have reported improvements using coconut oil in their children with autism, such as increased growth, fewer seizures, and improved behavior. Autism is actually a group of conditions known as autism spectrum disorders that appears to have many different causes, though largely unknown at present. Children with Down syndrome have an extra chromosome (47 instead of the normal 46), and the particular chromosome involved (chromosome 21) contains some of the genes that affect the development of Alzheimer's disease. Consequently, people with Down syndrome tend to develop Alzheimer's-type dementia as they enter middle age, with the characteristic plaques and tangles developing much earlier in life.

Studies using positron emission tomography (PET) scans, a unique type of imaging test that helps doctors identify abnormal from normal functioning of organs and tissues, have shown that some children with autism have decreased glucose uptake in certain areas of the brain. This is also true in some children and adults with Down syndrome, as well as in some children and adults with attention deficit disorders and bipolar disease. Therefore, ketones could potentially provide alternative fuel to the brains of children and adults with these conditions. During the Third International Symposium: Dietary Therapy for Epilepsy and Other Neurologic Disorders sponsored by the Charlie Foundation in Chicago in 2012, pediatrician Julie Buckley presented information about the use of a high-MCT-oil diet in children with autism. Her own daughter was normal up through age four, and then had an acute development of autism over several weeks, in which her speech regressed to that of an eighteen-month-old along with the development of severe behavior problems and seizures. Her daughter responded remarkably to a ketogenic diet that had a large portion of its calories as MCT oil, regaining 50 IQ points over about six months. Dr. Buckley has authored a book titled *Healing Our Autistic Children* (2010) and now specializes in helping families with autistic children in her practice near Jacksonville, Florida.

A reasonable amount of coconut oil to give a child would be to start with one-quarter teaspoon once or twice a day and gradually work up to one-quarter teaspoon of coconut oil for every ten pounds that the child weighs, three to four times a day, with food or in formula or milk. When that is tolerated, if desired, coconut oil can be further increased as tolerated. The total amount will vary greatly depending on the child's weight and ability to tolerate the oil without diarrhea. To give an idea of how much oil could be used in the diet for a child, there is a variation of the ketogenic diet, called the MCT oil–modified ketogenic diet, in which 60 percent of the calories in the diet are provided in the form of medium-chain triglycerides. This means that for every 1,000 calories, 600 calories come from medium-chain triglycerides, which equates to about six tablespoons of MCT oil or the equivalent amount of coconut oil. For parents of children with epilepsy or autism who wish to explore the use of a MCT oil–modified ketogenic diet, I highly recommend contacting the Charlie Foundation (www.charliefoundation.org) or Matthew's Friends (www.matthewsfriends.org) for guidance and referral to a dietitian highly experienced in helping families with ketogenic diets. As with our dietary guidelines here, these organizations generally recommend starting at a much lower percentage of MCT oil and increasing as tolerated to avoid diarrhea.

Also, some children like the taste of coconut milk, in which case the milk can be taken alone or added to other drinks. For coconut milk, I suggest adding one and one-half to two teaspoons to the diet for every ten pounds that the child weighs, two or three times a day. If you use coconut milk for a young child, be sure to refrigerate it and toss it after forty-eight hours. Do not add honey to coconut milk for children under one year old due to the risk of contamination with botulism. See the Coconut Milk recipes in Chapter 5 for suggested dilutions of canned coconut milk.

Can Coconut Oil Be Given to Animals?

One of the most unexpected e-mails I received was from a woman who wanted to know if coconut oil might improve cognition in her thirteen-year-old Welsh terrier. It is completely understandable that someone wouldn't want to see their beloved elderly pet suffer with dementia any more than another family member. It turns out that one of Accera's MCT-oil studies involved elderly dogs, and they did in fact show improved cognition in response to consuming the oil (Studzinski, 2008; Taha, 2009).

I relayed this information to her and suggested that she follow the guidelines for children: give one-quarter teaspoon for each ten pounds the dog weighs, two or three times a day. Her dog weighed twenty pounds, so she decided to give one-half teaspoon in her food twice a day. Several weeks later, she reported that her dog was getting up and around more, and finding her way to her food bowl, which she was not able to do prior to consuming the oil.

Dogs can also get diarrhea from coconut oil. The owner reported that one of her friends decided to use twice the recommended amount, and her dog developed diarrhea. Apparently, it is a good idea to start with caution and increase gradually with animals as well as people.

Since publication of my first book, I have heard from several other pet owners who feel their pets have improved while adding coconut oil to the diet. One family reported that their eight-year-old dog, a Havanese, that was diagnosed with epilepsy at age four and was not responding to a series of anticonvulsants, was seizure-free for more than four months after starting coconut and MCT oils in the diet and reducing carbohydrates. Ketogenic diets are not just for people and can be used in animals as well that have cancer, diabetes, weight issues, or other health problems. Just as in people, most of the processed foods manufactured for pets are considerably higher in carbohydrates than their pre-industrial era diet and include carbohydrates that they would never eat in the wild. A company called Ketopet (www.ketopet.com) can help with the ketogenic diet in animals.

What About Raspberry Ketones?

Many people have asked me whether raspberry ketones, which usually come in capsule form, have the same effect as the ketone ester or as ketones produced by consuming coconut oil or MCT oil. Raspberry ketones are artificially synthesized versions of the compound that causes the fruity aroma of red raspberries and are purported to burn fat. This ketone is a different molecule than the three naturally occurring ketones that are produced in the body and does not produce the same effect as far as providing alternative fuel to the brain. Even if raspberry ketone acted in this way, it would require dozens of capsules per day to provide the equivalent amount of energy.

How Can I Take Coconut Oil with Us When We Dine Out?

In this case, a single dose can be measured out, melted down, and placed into a small bottle, such as those in which food flavorings are packaged, or a 3-ounce travel bottle normally used for shampoo. One precaution: if you want to use plastic bottles, the safest type of plastic is polypropylene, since MCT oil will soften or split polyethylene and polystyrene. If there is no way to know what type of plastic the bottle is made from, then a small glass bottle would be the way to go. Most of the time, when melted down, the coconut oil will not become solid again for a couple of hours or longer, but if it does, the oil can be melted by placing it under warm running water in the restroom or in a cup of warm water, which the server would likely be happy to provide. I usually keep one or two doses for Steve in a resealable sandwich bag in my purse.

Another easy alternative would be to take along Fuel for Thought, which is packaged in small two-serving bottles that can be kept at room temperature for twenty-four hours after opening.

How Can We Continue This Dietary Intervention When Traveling?

Steve and I have faced this challenge a number of times, particularly on our long trips in 2010 to Greece and Scotland. I was quite worried at the time that we would have difficulty finding coconut oil and MCT oil when we arrived at our destination overseas or that Steve would miss doses while we were searching for them. Since we are currently limited when flying to several 3-ounce containers of gels and liquids in carry-on bags, I purchased small travel bottles normally used for shampoo and filled them with his mixture of coconut and MCT oils, which stays liquid at room temperature. Because certain plastics, such as polystyrene and polyethylene, but *not* polypropylene, can split or dissolve when in contact with MCT oil, it is a good idea to do your own test for this at home to make sure the container doesn't split or appear congealed.

To avoid the problem of what the bottles contained, I labeled them "Coconut/MCT Oil for Alzheimer's Patient." Each bottle contained two doses for Steve. I put the bottles into individual resealable sandwich bags and then placed all the bottles into a quart-size bag. This way if the contents leaked from one bottle, it would not ruin other items in the carry-on bag or purse. I packed enough of these bottles to give Steve all the doses he would need, plus a couple of extra doses; I did the same thing in the luggage, but in gallon-size bags. As an added precaution, I pack our clothes separately in huge 2x- and 3x-size resealable bags, available in the laundry section of our grocery store, and position the oil-containing bags in the suitcase so that they will not receive direct impact if the bag is thrown.

Another easy option now available is to take Fuel for Thought, which is packaged in two-serving bottles. I recommend placing the bottles inside at least one resealable bag.

Taking plain coconut oil in carry-on bags is a little trickier, as it tends to be solid at cooler temperatures and needs to be melted to get it into and out of the small travel bottles. One suggestion is to ask the flight attendant for a half-filled cup of warm water and then insert the bottle into the water cup. It should liquefy within five minutes. If that option is not available, try holding the container in your hand for a period of time, since body temperature is high enough to melt coconut oil. Some companies package their coconut oil in firm, tightly sealed plastic containers, which can be placed in a relatively protected section of the checked luggage, as described earlier. Again, I suggest placing the container in a resealable bag within another resealable bag.

We have had no difficulty to date taking our coconut oil and MCT oil with us while traveling using any of these methods.

What About Using Coconut Oil for Prevention?

People who have taken care of parents with dementias, Parkinson's disease, diabetes, and other such conditions are naturally worried that they may have witnessed their own future. Also, many notice as they age that their memory is not as sharp as it used to be and worry they are headed for Alzheimer's. Regular daily use of coconut oil or MCT oil or both could very well serve as a useful strategy for prevention.

An article was published in *Nutrition* in October 2011, titled "Brain Fuel Metabolism, Aging, and Alzheimer's Disease," by Stephen Cunnane, Ph.D., and his colleagues, who have done extensive studies on ketone metabolism at the University of Sherbrooke in Quebec using ketone-PET scanning, a new technology presently only available at this center. In the article the authors state, "Two observations in particular support the notion that the neurons affected in AD [Alzheimer's disease] are still functional: 1) in AD, brain ketone uptake is apparently normal or at least less impaired than is glucose; and 2) there is a functional response to nutritional supplements that increase brain fuel availability, particularly ketones. Hence, if brain fuel metabolism could be optimized or even partially returned toward normal, the risk of further cognitive decline may diminish. Raising plasma ketones to 0.4–0.5 millimoles per liter (mmol/L) would contribute from 5 to 10 percent of the brain's energy requirements, which is equivalent to the early cortical-glucose deficit in those genetically at risk [of] AD. Such a mild, safe level of ketonemia is achievable with ketogenic supplements, so if implemented before symptoms develop, it seems plausible that they could diminish the risk of further metabolic deterioration and clinical onset of cognitive decline" (Cunnane, 2011). Ketogenic supplements would include coconut oil, MCT oil, or a combination thereof.

New exciting work by Dr. Cunnane and his group, reported at the Clinical Trials Conference on Alzheimer's Disease in 2013 and published in 2015, demonstrates that, while the areas of the brain in people affected by Alzheimer's have abnormally low glucose uptake, these same areas have normal uptake of ketones comparable to that of healthy controls (Castellano, 2013 and 2015). This finding strongly supports the concept that ketones will provide alternative fuel to these glucose-deprived areas of the brain and would be useful to both treat and prevent this disease. The Alzheimer's Association has taken notice of this landmark study in ketone research and has awarded Dr. Cunnane a grant for a three-year study of the effects of MCT oil on cognition and the changes on ketone- and glucose-PET scanning in people with mild cognitive impairment, which often leads to Alzheimer's disease.

For those seeking prevention, I recommend beginning with one-half to one teaspoon of coconut oil or MCT oil, two or three times a day with food, and increasing this amount gradually to at least three to five tablespoons of coconut oil per day or, as an alternative, four teaspoons of MCT oil, three to four times a day with food. For myself, I average the equivalent of four to five tablespoons of coconut oil a day from a combination of coconut oil, MCT oil, coconut milk, and grated coconut. I also drink goat's milk instead of cow's milk, and enjoy feta or goat cheese on my salads since these contain medium-chain triglycerides as well.

Does Coconut Oil Have Other Benefits Besides Raising Ketones Levels?

Coconut oil is easily absorbed from the intestines and increases absorption of certain vitamins and minerals, and other important nutrients. This feature also holds true for coconut milk and coconut meat, whether wet or dry, such as unsweetened flaked or grated coconut. The fiber in coconut meat may be especially beneficial for people with Crohn's disease, other types of inflammatory bowel disease, or other malabsorption syndromes, and for people who have diarrhea from coconut or MCT oil.

All cell membranes and 60 to 70 percent of the brain are largely made up of fats. Many cell functions take place within the cell membrane. The majority of the fats that most of us consume today are vegetable oils, usually soybean or corn oil. These oils often contain hydrogenated and partially hydrogenated polyunsaturated fats and trans fats, which can carry potentially damaging oxygen-free radicals into cell membranes. Even non-hydrogenated polyunsaturated fatty acids can become oxidized (rancid) and pick up oxygen-free radicals. If you begin to substitute coconut and other natural oils, such as olive oil and even butter, along with omega-3 fatty acids in your meals, you may be able to undo some of the damage. Most of the cells in the body turn over within three to six months, and you may notice a nicer texture to your skin and a decrease in certain problems such as yeast and fungal infections.

Coconut oil is a wonderful moisturizer and personal lubricant, and is often used in tanning lotions and other skin-care products. In the tropics and areas where coconut oil is readily available, it is often applied to the skin before going out in the sun. Some people use coconut oil in their hair as a natural conditioner. Coconut oil feels soothing, is not sticky, and is absorbed readily into the skin. For dry skin, it can be applied while still damp after showering, and then lightly blotted dry.

A natural mixture to use as deodorant is to combine three tablespoons of coconut oil with one tablespoon each of corn powder and baking soda. The antimicrobial action of the lauric acid in coconut oil will kill bacteria that produce underarm odor.

Another somewhat surprising use for coconut oil is called "oil pulling," in which several teaspoons of coconut oil are worked around in the mouth and between the teeth for twenty minutes to effectively kill microorganisms and clean the teeth, reportedly an ancient practice. After a week or so of oil pulling, the teeth may feel as slick as they do following a cleaning by a dental hygienist. Using a toothbrush with coconut oil instead of the oil-pulling method produces surprisingly nice results, and adding a little baking soda to coconut oil may help whiten teeth as well.

For lengthy discussions of the many benefits of coconut oil, I highly recommend the books *Coconut Cures* (2005), *Oil Pulling Therapy* (2008), *Stop Alzheimer's Now* (2011), and *The Coconut Oil Miracle* (2013), all by Bruce Fife, N.D.

4

More About MCT Oil
with Questions and Answers

When I was doing my pediatric residency and fellowship training in neonatology in the late 1970s and early 1980s, it was a standard practice to add medium-chain triglyceride oil, also known as MCT oil, to the feedings of our smallest premature newborns. They were known to digest the oil easily and it would effectively help them gain weight and get home sooner. Little did we know that this strategy may have provided some neuroprotection as well. Theodore VanItallie, M.D., and Sami Hashim, M.D., pioneers in nutrition and metabolism research, along with their associates, studied MCT oil extensively beginning in the 1960s in both children and adults, defining some of its important properties, including its easy absorption from the bowel and partial conversion to ketones in the liver (Bergen, 1966). Today, virtually every infant formula in the United States contains MCT oil, coconut oil, and/or palm kernel oil. Medium-chain triglycerides are found in human breast milk and are added to infant formulas largely for this reason. Many liquid nutritional supplements for bodybuilders and for undernourished adults contain MCT oil as well.

In May 2008 when I was researching on the Internet the risks and benefits of two drugs about to begin clinical trials that Steve might qualify for, I happened purely by chance upon a press release discussing a new medical food in development called AC-1202. The product improved memory and cognition in nearly half the people who received it in their clinical trials, compared to the placebo (Reger, 2004; Henderson, 2008). The press release did not say exactly what it was or how it worked, but, digging further, I found the patent application for the product and soon learned that the only active ingredient was caprylic triglyceride, a type of MCT oil. Furthermore, I learned that MCT oil is extracted from coconut oil or palm kernel oil. It was because of my personal experience as a pediatrician and neonatologist with MCT oil that I recognized the potential for this treatment.

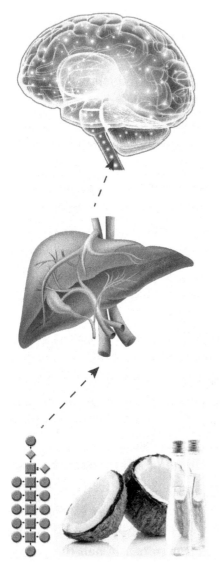

The patent application for AC-1202 discussed at length the concept of Alzheimer's disease as type 3 diabetes, or diabetes of the brain, a concept that was new to me. It also reminded me of information I had learned in medical school Biochemistry 101: that ketones are an alternative fuel for the brain during starvation and, that, when consumed, MCT oil is partly converted to ketones in the liver. See Figure 4.1.

FIGURE 4.1. MCT oil is absorbed from the intestines and taken directly to the liver where part of it is converted to ketones. The remaining MCTs are released in the bloodstream and are used immediately as fuel in mitochondria of muscles, the brain, and other organs.

As mentioned previously, it's a common misconception that all saturated fats are bad and are to be avoided. Not only is this excessive fear of saturated fat unwarranted, but, far from detrimental, medium-chain triglycerides are saturated fats with special properties that may actually provide health benefits. These fatty acids are not found in significant amounts in the typical low-fat, high-carb Western diet.

Before talking about the very special nature of MCT oil, a crash course on fatty acids might be helpful.

FATTY ACIDS

Fats, also known as lipids, are comprised of triglycerides, which consist of three fatty acid molecules combined with a glycerol molecule. There are two major ways of classifying fatty acids: one, by the length of the fatty acid chain; and the other, by how saturated the chain is with hydrogen atoms.

Fatty acids consist of chains of carbon atoms attached to one another, end to end, much like railroad train cars. On either side of each carbon is a site that can be occupied by a hydrogen atom. At one end of the chain, the carbon atom has an additional hydrogen atom attached to it. At the other end of the chain, the carbon atom is attached to an oxygen atom and a hydroxyl molecule, which is comprised of an oxygen atom and a hydrogen atom.

Fatty acids are further classified as short-, medium-, long- and very-long-chain fatty acids, depending on how many carbon atoms are in the chain. A short-chain fatty acid has less than six carbons in the chain; a medium-chain fatty acid has six to twelve carbons; a long-chain fatty acid, fourteen to twenty-two carbons; and a very-long-chain fatty acid, more than twenty-two carbons. The length of the carbon chain affects the various properties of each fatty acid.

Short- and medium-chain fatty acids are digested faster and more easily than long-chain and very-long-chain fatty acids. They do not require bile acids and are absorbed from the bowel and taken directly to the liver by way of the portal vein (a blood vessel that conducts blood from the gastrointestinal tract to the liver and spleen). In the liver, some of these fatty acids are converted to ketones, which can be used an alternative fuel to glucose in all organs except the liver where they are made, and some are released directly into the circulation to be delivered to other tissues and used directly by mitochondria to produce energy.

Short-chain fatty acids are found in milk fat and are also produced in small quantities in the colon when fiber is fermented. Medium-chain fatty acids are only produced in the body as a component of breast milk in the mammary glands of lactating women (Bitman, 1983). After weaning, medium-chain fatty acids must come from food and are mainly found in coconut oil, palm kernel oil, and in the milk fat of other mammals, particularly in goats and to a lesser degree in cows. MCT oil is usually extracted from coconut or palm kernel oil.

Long- and very-long-chain fatty acids require bile salts and enzymes called lipases to be broken apart prior to their absorption from the intestines. After absorption, they are repackaged as triglycerides and carried throughout the body by way of the lymphatic system as chylomicrons (lipoproteins), globules of fats, and proteins. Little or no ketone is produced from these longer-chain fatty acids in the person consuming a typical diet. Most naturally occurring vegetable and animal fats consist primarily of long- and very-long-chain fatty acids.

In addition to the length of the carbon chain, the second way of classifying fatty acids is by how saturated the carbon chain is with hydrogen atoms at the available sites adjacent to the carbon atoms. There are three major categories of fatty acids—saturated, monounsaturated, and polyunsaturated. With the exception of the first and last carbon in the chain, each carbon atom has two sites potentially available for a hydrogen atom to form a bond with it.

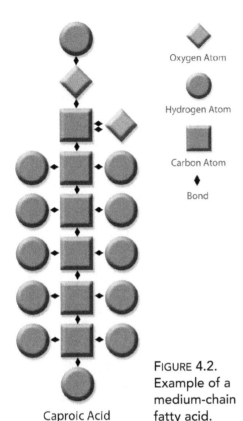

Caproic Acid

Oxygen Atom

Hydrogen Atom

Carbon Atom

Bond

FIGURE 4.2.
Example of a
medium-chain
fatty acid.

In a saturated fatty acid, all the potential sites along the carbon chain are occupied by hydrogen atoms. A mono-unsaturated fatty acid has a single site where two adjacent carbon atoms are each missing a hydrogen atom, and these two carbon atoms then form a stronger double bond between then. Atoms or molecules other than hydrogen can attach to these double-bond sites. A polyunsaturated fatty acid has more than one of these double-bond sites. (See Figures 4.2 and 4.3.)

All medium-chain fatty acids are saturated fats, which tend to be very stable and do not spoil easily at room temperature, resulting in a very long shelf life. Some long- and very-long-chain fatty acids are saturated, some are monounsaturated, and some are polyunsaturated. The more unsaturated a fat is, the quicker it can spoil, or become rancid, as a result of oxidation. Oxidation is a process in which fats, left exposed or subjected to heat sources, interact with oxygen and create oxygen-free radicals. Oxygen-free radicals, also called oxidants or reactive oxygen species, are natural byproducts of some chemical reactions in the body and may serve a purpose, but, when released and present in excess, can cause damage to cells and tissues.

Olive oil is an example of a predominantly monounsaturated fat and soybean oil is a predominantly polyunsaturated fat. Omega-3 and omega-6 fatty acids are examples of polyunsaturated fatty

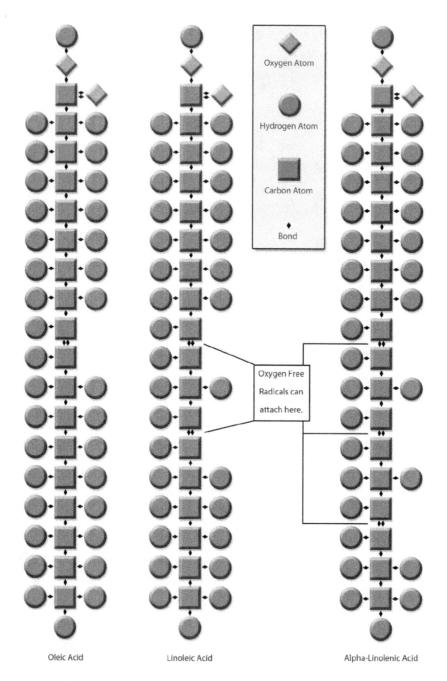

Oxygen Atom

Hydrogen Atom

Carbon Atom

Bond

Oxygen Free
Radicals can
attach here.

Oleic Acid   Linoleic Acid   Alpha-Linolenic Acid

FIGURE 4.3. Examples of a monounsaturated fatty acid (left)
and two polyunsaturated fatty acids (middle and right).

acids. There are varying chain lengths of omega-3 and omega-6 fatty acids. The omega number refers to where the first double-bond site occurs in relation to the end of the molecule; for instance, if the first double bond is at the third carbon from the end of the chain, it is an omega-3 fatty acid.

There is a misconception that commonly used oils for cooking contain no saturated fats, but, in fact, they do. Most naturally occurring vegetable and animal fats and oils contain a combination of saturated, monounsaturated, and polyunsaturated fatty acids of varying chain lengths. For example, the saturated fat content in soybean oil is 15.6 percent; olive oil, 13.8 percent; corn oil, 13.0 percent; and canola oil, 7.4 percent. Similarly, the fat beneath the skin (subcutaneous fat) also contains a combination of fats and is roughly 27 percent saturated, 50 percent monounsaturated, and 23 percent polyunsaturated fatty acids give or take a few percent in either direction depending on the diet (Ren, 2008).

Special Properties of Medium-Chain Fatty Acids

To keep the discussion simple, in this section we will use the abbreviation based on the number of carbons in the chain of the medium-chain triglyceride. Table 4.1 (on page 128) shows the common abbreviations and names for the four basic medium-chain triglycerides as well as their chemical structures.

Coconut oil is the richest natural source of medium-chain triglycerides, containing up to 60 percent, followed by palm kernel oil. Medium-chain fatty acids are also present in the milk fat of humans and other mammals, particularly in goat's milk and to a lesser degree in cow's milk. In contrast, there are no medium-chain triglycerides in other commonly used oils, such as olive, soybean, canola, safflower, and fish oil. MCT oil is a man-made product that is usually extracted from coconut or palm kernel oil. Most over-the-counter brands of MCT oil contain a formulation that is prima-

TABLE 4.1. THE MEDIUM-CHAIN TRIGLYCERIDES

ABBREVIATION BASED ON # OF CARBON ATOMS IN CHAIN	CHEMICAL STRUCTURE	COMMON NAMES
C:6	$CH_3(CH_2)_4COOH$	CAPROIC ACID; HEXANOIC ACID
C:8	$CH_3(CH_2)_6COOH$	CAPRYLIC ACID; OCTANOIC ACID
C:10	$CH_3(CH_2)_8COOH$	CAPRIC ACID; DECANOIC ACID
C:12	$CH_3(CH_2)_{10}COOH$	LAURIC ACID; DODECANOIC ACID

rily C:8, and then C:10, with minimal amounts of C:6 and C:12. However, it is possible to buy almost pure C:8 MCT oil over the counter (see Resources section). This formulation is relevant because C:8 is caprylic triglyceride, the active ingredient in medical food Axona. C:8 is thought to be the most ketogenic of the medium-chain triglycerides, meaning that more of it is converted to ketones in the liver before it is released into the general circulation.

There are a several differences between medium-chain triglycerides and longer-chain triglycerides that result in significant health advantages from consuming the medium-chain fatty acids. Along with their easy digestibility, medium-chain triglycerides appear to enhance absorption of other substances such as calcium, magnesium, and amino acids, potentially providing a nutritional advantage for those who have an immature bowel, such as a premature newborn, and people with impaired fat metabolism and malabsorption syndromes, such as biliary cirrhosis, Crohn's disease, regional enteritis, celiac disease, or pancreatitis (Tantibhehyangkul, 1975; Sulkers, 1992; Shea, 2003; Cabre, 2012).

Also, unlike long-chain triglycerides, medium-chain fatty acids easily pass through the cell membrane and into the mitochondria where energy is made without enzymes or a shuttle system. Once inside the mitochondria, they enter the complex metabolic pathways ultimately used to make ATP or are further converted to ketones. Medium-chain triglycerides are used directly to make energy in skeletal and cardiac muscle, and are also taken up by the mitochondria in astrocytes, special brain cells that provide nutrition to the neurons, where they are also partly converted to ketones (Auestad, 1991). So in this sense, medium-chain triglycerides provide another source of alternative fuel to the brain, which could at least partly explain why consumption of these fatty acids can produce such dramatic improvement in some people, in spite of the relatively small increase in ketone levels that occurs.

Medium-chain triglycerides provide about 8.3 calories per gram compared with 9.0 calories for long-chain triglycerides, and because these fatty acids are converted directly to fuel for immediate use, they are not stored as fat. For this reason, they are useful for people who have increased energy needs, such as those recovering from surgery, severe injuries or burns, or dealing with cancer and cancer treatments. Medium-chain fatty acids also have been shown to increase physical endurance, and, coupled with the increased immediate energy availability, would be useful to those who desire to enhance their athletic performance, as well as to the elderly or frail who wish to have more energy.

In addition, compared to long-chain triglycerides, medium-chain fatty acids are relatively thermogenic, which means that they increase metabolic rate and therefore more calories are burned over twenty-four hours. A number of studies in animals and people have shown that, when equivalent amounts of either medium-chain triglycerides or long-chain triglycerides are added to the diet, or when a high-fat diet rich in medium-chain triglycerides is eaten, compared to a low-fat diet, much less fat is deposited by those consuming the high-MCT oil diet. Also, medium-chain triglycerides appear to suppress appetite, resulting in fewer calories consumed. The net result is that a diet rich in these fatty acids could be useful as a weight-loss or weight-maintenance strategy, as long as they are substituted for other fats and/or carbohydrates in the diet and are not simply added to the existing diet.

Another unique property of medium-chain triglycerides is that they significantly increase the use of glucose in cells, which is mediated by insulin (both in diabetics and non-diabetics), thereby potentially providing improved glucose control in the diabetic and in people with other conditions complicated by insulin resistance, such as Alzheimer's and Parkinson's disease. It could be then that another reason medium-chain triglycerides may improve memory and cognition is that they enhance the uptake of glucose in the brain.

One experiment that highlights the neuroprotective effects of medium-chain triglycerides was reported by Kathleen Page, M.D., and others in *Diabetes* (Page, 2009). The subjects of this study were brittle type 1 diabetics, a term used to describe diabetics who have great difficulty controlling their blood glucose levels and are prone to repeated episodes of hypoglycemia (low blood sugar) with attendant clouding of thought processes. Most of the individuals in the study were using insulin pumps to control their blood sugar. Each person served as his or her own control, receiving MCT oil on one occasion and a placebo on another, and each was given enough insulin to deliberately cause hypoglycemia. When the participants received the placebo, they had significant deterioration in their scores on several cognitive tests, but, remarkably, this did not occur when they received the MCT oil. The bottom line here is that including medium-chain triglycerides in the diet of the diabetic may help counter some of the effects of low-blood sugar episodes. It could, for example, be helpful for a diabetic to take MCT oil before retiring for the night if that is a common time for the person to have an attack of low blood sugar. In addition, certain complications of diabetes, such as kidney and retinal damage, are likely a result of insulin resistance (Svensson, 2006) and potentially could be lessened by regularly consuming ketone-producing medium-chain triglycerides.

There are yet other properties of medium-chain triglycerides that appear to be beneficial to health. As just one example, lauric acid (C:12) is known to have antimicrobial effects against various yeast, protozoa, and bacteria, such as *Helicobacter pylori,* which causes ulcers and is more common in brains of people with Alzheimer's. Lauric acid has even been shown to dissolve the lipid capsule, enveloping herpes and HIV viruses; the herpes simplex virus has been implicated as well as a possible cause of Alzheimer's in some people. Lauric acid is one of the components of breast milk that is believed to protect the newborn from infection with abnormal organisms and at the same time to support the growth of normal gut bacteria (Isaacs, 1994; Isaacs, 1995). When used to support the immune system against microorganisms, coconut oil, which is roughly 50 percent lauric acid, may be preferable to MCT oil.

Stephen Cunnane, Ph.D., and his associates in Canada have learned from glucose- and ketone-PET scans and other types of studies that use of ketones by the brain does not appear to be affected by aging or by Alzheimer's disease, but is somewhat lower in diabetics. They have also learned that areas of the brain where there is decreased glucose uptake in people with mild Alzheimer's appear to take up ketones normally (Castellano, 2015). This important finding would seem to support a hypothesis that the decrease in glucose uptake may not simply be a result of dead neurons, but rather that there are viable cells lying dormant in these areas of the brain for which ketones could provide alternative fuel. The researchers have also discovered that the plasma concentration of ketones is directly proportional to the percent of energy supplied by ketones to the brain. Thus, a ketone level of 0.4 to 0.5 mmol/L, which can be achieved by taking medium-chain fatty acids, could provide 5 to 10 percent of the brain's energy needs, which is equivalent to the deficit in energy provided to the brain by glucose in people who are genetically at risk for Alzheimer's (Cunnane, 2011).

ds, regular consumption of coconut or MCT oil or
entially provide a nutritional prevention strategy to
sk of developing Alzheimer's, or at least delay onset
. Ketone esters and salts, currently in development,
can easily produce levels many times higher than MCT oil and
therefore would be expected to provide substantially more energy
to the brain. Until these ketone products are available on the market, coconut and/or MCT oil use is a reasonable, albeit likely a less
effective, alternative.

QUESTIONS AND ANSWERS ABOUT MCT OIL

I knew for several decades that MCT oil existed, since it was in use
in newborn intensive care units as early as the 1970s. I assumed it
was only available to hospitals, but not long after Steve responded
to coconut oil, I learned that it could easily be purchased over the
counter. I was surprised to find it in several local natural food stores
and to learn that it is commonly used by bodybuilders to increase
lean body mass. Following are the most frequently asked questions
I receive about using MCT oil.

What Is Over-the-Counter MCT Oil?

MCT oil is usually derived from coconut oil or palm kernel oil.
Medium-chain fatty acids are prepared commercially by breaking
down coconut oil (and sometimes palm kernel oil) into its individual components (called hydrolysis). The medium-chain fatty acids
are then separated from the longer-chain fatty acids by steam distil-
lation. The medium-chain fatty acids, which are quite acidic and
inedible as such, are then recombined with glycerol to make the
medium-chain triglycerides for consumption.

Most over-the-counter MCT products are a mixture of triglycerides—predominantly caprylic (C:8), some capric (C:10), and small amounts of caproic (C:6) and lauric acids (C:12)—the four medium-chain triglycerides found in coconut oil. Coconut oil, which is about 60 percent medium-chain fatty acids, contains a much larger proportion of lauric acid than MCT oil. There is much ado about how high coconut oil is in saturated fats, however, about 70 percent of the saturated fats in coconut oil are medium-chain fatty acids, which behave very differently than long-chain saturated fats as discussed earlier in this section. One brand of MCT oil, called CapTri, from Parrillo Performance (www.parrillo.com), is approximately 97 percent tri-caprylic acid, the active ingredient in the medical food Axona (discussed shortly). Four teaspoons (20 grams) of this MCT oil is equivalent to one dose of Axona. The company also offers butter-flavored MCT oil, as well as a number of other food products that contain MCT oil.

MCT oil can be used as an alternative to coconut oil to produce mild ketosis. The primary differences between using MCT oil and coconut oil are that a smaller volume of MCT oil can be taken without the additional fatty acids found in coconut oil, and that the levels of ketones may be higher, although compared to coconut oil they tend to leave the circulation after a few hours.

The Japanese company Nisshin Oillio (mentioned earlier) has created a product called Healthy Resetta Oil, which contains a special MCT oil with a long-chain triglyceride attached to the compound that results in a better oil for cooking at higher heat without foaming yet that retains the healthy property of MCT oil. The company also makes powdered MCT oil and is constantly developing new food products that contain MCT oil, such as salad oils, mayonnaise, and fruit-flavored puddings.

Another company called True Protein (www.trueprotein.com) offers a nonprescription powdered form of MCT oil combined with some carbohydrate that can be added to liquids or pureed foods, or added to recipes.

est Way to Store MCT Oil?

:ns or splits certain plastics such as polyethylene and ›ut not polypropylene. If you are unsure that the plastic containɛ you wish to store it in is made of polypropylene, it is recommended that MCT oil be stored in glass, metal, or ceramic containers (Sucher, 1986).

Someone recently advised me that she had mixed MCT oil into coffee in a Styrofoam cup and forgot to drink it. When she returned she noticed that the cup had been partly dissolved. Since I wasn't sure whether it was the MCT oil specifically or a combination of the hot coffee and MCT oil, I performed a little experiment, placing room-temperature MCT oil alone in a cup, and also MCT oil and coffee in another cup. In the MCT-oil-only cup, the oil leached through the bottom of the cup; in the cup with the MCT oil and coffee, the mixture leached through and minute droplets of coffee and oil appeared on the outside of the cup. The take-home message here is to use a ceramic or glass cup when adding MCT oil to a liquid to drink, whether hot or cold.

How Can I Avoid Diarrhea?

The most common complaint with MCT oil is the problem of diarrhea, which usually occurs if too much oil is taken by someone who has not taken it before or if the amount of oil is increased too quickly. MCT oil is more likely than coconut oil to produce this problem, which occurs in about 25 percent of people as they begin taking the oil. On the other hand, some people report to me that they have a greater problem with coconut oil than MCT oil. Considering the amount of oil that one may consume in a day's time— upward of six to eight tablespoons or more—most people will find the level at which they have diarrhea, which usually happens within an hour or so of eating the oil. An occasional person will experience diarrhea with just one teaspoon, so caution should be exercised with the first dose.

The following strategies help decrease the likelihood of developing diarrhea:

1. Start with a small amount of oil, such as one-half to one teaspoon once or twice a day, and increase slowly as tolerated. Increase by one teaspoon every few days until reaching the desired amount, possibly as much as two or more tablespoons, three to four times a day.

2. Always take the oil with other foods.

3. Take the oil slowly during the course of a meal, over twenty to thirty minutes. If the oil is mixed with food, this will be easier to accomplish.

4. Mixing the oil with cottage cheese may decrease the odds that diarrhea will occur, so it might be practical to take the oil with cottage cheese one or more times per day. Cottage cheese is also an excellent source of protein and provides a relatively small amount of carbohydrate.

5. If using even small amounts of oil persists in causing diarrhea, consider trying other coconut products such as coconut milk or even grated coconut, which contains a substantial amount of MCT oil. The oil may be released more slowly in the course of digestion and therefore be less likely to set off diarrhea.

6. If a person cannot tolerate coconut oil or MCT oil in any form, consideration should be given to massaging coconut oil into the skin, as it gets absorbed quickly and well. One caregiver reported that her mother improved with coconut oil, but that it gave her diarrhea even with very small amounts and had to be discontinued. The daughter saw the improvements in her mother disappear. However, after she began massaging her

mother's skin with coconut oil, she saw the improvements return once again. In addition, several people with ALS have been using coconut oil as a massage over weakened muscles and believe they have experienced benefits from it, including increased measurement around the thigh by several centimeters (inches). (To read more about these personal accounts, see Chapter 10.)

This idea may have some scientific validity, in that a study at the Garvan Institute of Medical Research in Australia by Nigel Turner, Ph.D., and others using coconut oil found that medium-chain triglycerides enter the mitochondria of muscle cells directly (Turner, 2009). In addition, some bodybuilders claim that massaging coconut oil over sore muscles may reduce the pain. In one review of infant-massage therapy studies, it was reported that premature infants massaged with coconut or safflower oil gained weight faster, had increased bone density, and left the neonatal intensive care unit sooner than infants who did not receive this massage. In addition, there was a measurable increase in triglycerides in the blood after the massage with these oils, confirming that these oils are absorbed through the skin (Field, 2010). If coconut and MCT oils result in diarrhea no matter how it is consumed, massage may be worth trying.

7. A possible alternative to using MCT oil for those who cannot tolerate or are allergic to it is to take another type of compound that might serve as an alternative fuel. One of these compounds is alpha-ketoglutarate, a substance used by bodybuilders to improve peak athletic performance. It is available in several different powder and pill forms. Alpha-ketoglutarate is one of the key intermediates further down the pathway in the same chain of events that ketones can fuel, leading ultimately to synthesis of the energy molecule ATP.

Alpha-ketoglutarate came to light as a possible treatment for neurodegenerative disorders as the result of research by Vince

Tedone, M.D., a retired orthopedic surgeon in Tampa, Florida, whose daughter Deanna has ALS and uses alpha-ketoglutarate. She also receives massages with coconut oil and takes coconut oil with her food. She has had minimal worsening over nearly three years with this approach, called the Deanna Protocol. Information about how ketosis and alpha-ketoglutarate may reduce nerve cell death is available on their website at www. winningthefight.net. The amount that will produce results is unknown at this time but their website suggests a minimum of 2 to 6 grams (2,000–6,000 mg) per day with some people slowly working up to 12 to 18 grams (12,000–18,000 mg) per day. Alpha-ketoglutyrate is available in several different powder and pill forms. Their foundation, called Winning the Fight, is funding clinical studies on the use of the Deana protocol in ALS models of mice currently in progress at the University of South Florida and already is showing promising results (Ari, 2014). Clinical trials in people with ALS will follow.

What Is Axona?

For those who prefer a method to take medium-chain triglycerides prescribed and monitored by their physician, Axona, a medical food from the Accera Company, is available. This is a powdered form of MCT oil (specifically caprylic triglyceride) mixed with some other nutrients and emulsifiers that dissolve in liquids and can be taken as a drink. Current recommendations are to take Axona once a day in the morning. The initial pilot study of 20 people and follow-up phase II studies of 152 people taking Axona (then called AC-1202) versus a placebo are described in detail in my previous book. In each of these studies, more than 40 percent of the people had significant cognitive improvement (Reger, 2004; Costantini, 2008). In both studies, the group of people who were negative for the ApoE4 gene improved on average and those who were positive for this gene as a group did not, however, some individuals with the ApoE4 gene did improve.

More recently a retrospective study was reported of fifty-five patients at eleven different physician practices who were diagnosed with probable mild to moderate Alzheimer's disease and received caprylic triglyceride (as Axona) for at least six months. They found that about 80 percent of the patients who added caprylic triglyceride to their ongoing pharmacologic treatment were stable or improved on their physician's overall assessment after eighteen months, and their Mini-Mental Status Exam scores remained stable over fifteen months of therapy. Likewise, 80 percent improved or remained stable according to caregiver assessments of their ability to perform various activities at home and recognition of family members over this same time frame. The only adverse effects reported were gastrointestinal (Maynard, 2013). The same authors published a series of eight case reports selected from these fifty-five patients to represent the various responses to Axona that were seen in this study (Maynard, 2013).

A study of more frequent dosing with Axona is in progress as of this writing, but currently the company is bound by FDA rules to recommend just the once-a-day dosing they used in their studies to obtain FDA approval. For more information, go to www.about-axona.com. A very helpful video demonstrating how ketones work as an alternative fuel is available at the site.

Why Do You Mix MCT Oil and Coconut Oil?

About two months after starting Steve on coconut oil and receiving results of his ketone levels, we began experimenting with mixing MCT oil and coconut oil. When Steve took just coconut oil in the morning, his ketone levels peaked at about three hours and were nearly gone after eight to nine hours, just before dinner time. Steve's ketone levels with just MCT oil were higher but gone within three hours. I reasoned that a mixture of MCT oil and coconut oil should result in higher levels and longer-lasting levels, and that if Steve was given this mixture three to four times a day, some ketones would always be circulating and available to his brain.

Why Not Use Just MCT Oil?

If you decide to take just MCT oil several times a day, the levels fluctuate up and down more than with coconut oil or with a mixture of coconut and MCT oils. Also, some fatty acids in whole coconut oil are not found in MCT oil, and I believe that they might contribute to the improvements seen in Steve and others. For example, the lauric acid in coconut oil kills certain types of viruses, such as those that cause fever blisters. At least one group of researchers has found evidence of the herpes simplex virus type 1 that causes fever blisters in the beta-amyloid plaques in the brains of people with Alzheimer's, especially those with the ApoE4 gene like Steve (Wozniak, 2010).

Taking coconut oil seems to be helpful for Steve in that he was regularly fighting fever blisters, sometimes for several weeks at a time. These episodes have become less severe and less frequent, with just four episodes over the past six years. These fever-blister outbreaks have coincided with other infections and new medication-related setbacks, adding more weight to the idea that this virus may contribute to the progression of Alzheimer's disease.

Why Not Use Just Coconut Oil?

Many people have reported to me that they have seen improvements in their loved ones with Alzheimer's using just coconut oil. Steve had a dramatic improvement using just coconut oil for the first two months. I don't know for certain whether there is any additional benefit to adding MCT oil, so I see no problem with using just coconut oil for this dietary intervention. One reason to consider adding MCT oil would be to achieve higher levels of ketones. In the Axona (MCT oil) studies, people with higher levels tended to have more improvement in cognitive function. Because only part of MCT oil is converted to ketones, the remaining medium-chain fatty acids could potentially be used by neurons as an alternative fuel—and the more MCT oil one can tolerate, the more ketones and medium-chain triglycerides will be available to the brain. Much more needs to be learned about what medium-chain fatty acids exactly do.

Another point to consider is that by mixing MCT oil and coconut oil in a four-to-three ratio, the long-chain saturated fatty acids are reduced to 10 percent of the total fat. Recent studies are finding less and less evidence that saturated fat and cholesterol are the culprits in heart disease. But for those who are still worried about the possible health issues related to saturated fats, this mixture of MCT and coconut oils offers an alternative to using an equivalent amount of just coconut oil.

## 5

Recipes: Cooking with Coconut and MCT Oils

Here are some of the recipes that we use in our home to enjoy coconut oil and MCT oil in our diet.

ESSENTIAL STARTERS

MCT AND COCONUT OIL 4:3 MIXTURE

YIELD: 28 ounces

• •

16 ounces MCT oil

12 ounces coconut oil

Directions: Warm the coconut oil until it is completely liquid by placing the container in a pan of hot water. Use a funnel to add the MCT and coconut oils to a glass quart container such as a MCT oil bottle, then cap it securely and invert it several times to mix the oils. Shake before each use. Store at room temperature.

Optional: Add 1 or more tablespoons of liquid soy lecithin to allow for easier mixing with other liquids.

THIN-STYLE COCONUT MILK

YIELD: Each 6.5 ounces provides 15 grams
(about 1 tablespoon) of coconut oil

• •

1 can undiluted full-fat coconut milk (with 11 grams fat per 2 ounces)

1$\frac{1}{2}$ cans of water or coconut water

10 drops liquid stevia or 1 to 2 teaspoons of honey, agave syrup,
or other sweetener to taste

Pinch of salt

Directions: Place the ingredients in a container and shake well before use. Store the coconut milk in the refrigerator and discard the unused portion after four days. When used for children, discard the coconut milk after two days.

Variation: Add 1 of teaspoon dolomite powder to the mixture to supplement the diet with additional calcium and magnesium.

THICK-STYLE COCONUT MILK

YIELD: Each 4 ounces provides 15 grams
(about 1 tablespoon) of coconut oil

• •

1 can undiluted full-fat coconut milk (with 11 grams fat per 2 ounces)

$\frac{1}{2}$ can water or coconut water

10 drops liquid stevia or 1 to 2 teaspoons of honey, agave syrup,
or other sweetener to taste

Pinch of salt

Directions: Place the ingredients in a container and shake well before use. Store the coconut milk in the refrigerator and discard the unused portion after four days. When used for children, discard the coconut milk after two days.

Variation: Add 1 teaspoon of dolomite powder to the mixture to supplement the diet with additional calcium and magnesium.

MCT SKIM MILK

YIELD: One 4- to 8-ounce serving

. . . .

4 to 8 ounces skim milk

Your usual serving of MCT oil or MCT/
Coconut Oil 4:3 Mixture (page 141)

Directions: Place the milk in a glass. Add the MCT oil or MCT and coconut oil mixture and stir thoroughly together with a small wire whisk or fork.

BREAKFASTS
TO GREET YOUR DAY

ORANGE-COCONUT MILK

YIELD: One 8- to 10-ounce serving

. . . .

4 to 6 ounces Thick-Style Coconut Milk (page 142),
Thin-Style Coconut Milk (page 142), or cow's or goat's milk
while gradually increasing your coconut oil intake

4 ounces orange juice or diet orange soda

Extra coconut oil (melted) or MCT and Coconut Oil 4:3 Mixture
(page 141) (optional)

Directions: Place the milk in a 12-ounce glass, then slowly add the orange juice or diet orange soda, and the coconut oil or the MCT and coconut mixture if using. Mix thoroughly with a spoon.

Variation: Try diet grape soda or diet root beer instead of orange soda.

COCONUT MILK QUICK PROTEIN DRINK

YIELD: One 8-ounce serving

• •

2 tablespoons whey, rice, pea, or egg-white protein powder
or combination of these

1 cup Thin-Style Coconut Milk (page 142)

Extra coconut oil (melted) or MCT and Coconut Oil 4:3 Mixture
(page 141) (optional)

Directions: Place the protein powder in the coconut milk and mix thoroughly
with a wire whisk until dissolved.

BERRY-COCONUT MILK SMOOTHIE

YIELD: One 14- to 16-ounce serving

• •

$1/2$ cup crushed ice

1 cup frozen blueberries or 4 large frozen strawberries

$1/3$ cup bran cereal (such as Fiber One Original or Smart Bran)
or equivalent of sliced almonds (a lower carb choice)

1 teaspoon honey, agave syrup, or equivalent sweetener such as stevia

1 cup Thick-Style Coconut Milk (page 142), Thin-Style Coconut Milk (page 142),

or cow's or goat's milk while gradually increasing your coconut oil intake

1 egg, hard-boiled or raw

2 tablespoons vanilla-flavored or unflavored whey protein powder

Extra coconut oil (melted) or MCT and Coconut Oil
4:3 Mixture (page 141) (optional)

Directions: Place all the ingredients in a blender, add the coconut oil or the
MCT/coconut oil mixture if using, and process for about 30 seconds until
smooth and creamy. If the mixture is too thick, add more milk as needed.

Note: For those who are concerned about adding raw egg, microwave the egg for about 20 seconds to kill bacteria before adding to other ingredients.

Variations: Add $1/_2$ banana and 2 large strawberries per serving or substitute an equivalent amount of apple, blueberry, or pomegranate juice for part or all of the milk.

COCONUT-EGG-HIGH-PROTEIN PROBIOTIC SMOOTHIE

YIELD: One 12- to 14-ounce serving

• •

3 eggs, hard-boiled or raw

2 tablespoons vanilla-flavored or unflavored whey protein

10 to 15 drops liquid stevia

4 ounces plain whole-fat kefir

4 to 6 ounces Thick-Style Coconut Milk (page 142),
Thin-Style Coconut Milk (page 142),
or cow's or goat's milk while gradually increasing
your coconut oil intake

Extra coconut oil (melted) or MCT and Coconut Oil 4:3 Mixture
(page 141) (optional)

Directions: Combine all the ingredients in a blender, add the coconut oil or the MCT/coconut oil mixture if using, and blend until mixed well.

Note: Adding kefir (a fermented milk with active cultures) is a great way to incorporate probiotics in to the diet. For those who are concerned about adding raw egg, microwave the eggs for about 20 seconds to kill any bacteria before adding to the other ingredients.

Variations: Add one of the following: several cut-up fresh or fresh frozen strawberries, $1/_2$ cup of blueberries, 2 ounces of fruit or green liquid smoothie, 2 teaspoons of cherry juice concentrate, or 1 to 2 tablespoons of Earth Balance Coconut and Peanut Spread.

BANANA-PEANUT BUTTER-COCONUT MILK SMOOTHIE

YIELD: One 14- to 16-ounce serving

· ·

$1/2$ cup crushed ice

1 frozen banana (break into four pieces before freezing)

$1/3$ cup bran cereal (such as Fiber One Original or Smart Bran)
or equivalent of sliced almonds (a lower carb choice)

1 tablespoon fresh ground or natural peanut
or almond butter

1 teaspoon honey, agave syrup,
or equivalent sweetener such as stevia

1 cup Thick-Style Coconut Milk (page 142),
Thin-Style Coconut Milk (page 142),
or cow's or goat's milk while gradually increasing
your coconut oil intake

1 egg, hard-boiled or raw

2 tablespoons vanilla flavored or unflavored
whey protein powder

Extra coconut oil (melted) or MCT and
Coconut Oil 4:3 Mixture (page 141) (optional)

Directions: Place all the ingredients in a blender, add the coconut oil or the MCT/coconut mixture if using, and process for about 30 seconds until smooth and creamy. If the mixture is too thick, add more coconut milk as needed.

Note: For those who are concerned about using raw egg, microwave the egg for about 20 seconds to kill the bacteria before adding to other ingredients.

GREEN COCONUT SMOOTHIE

YIELD: One 14- to 16-ounce serving

$^1/_2$ cup crushed ice

$^1/_3$ cup sliced almonds (optional)

1 cup leafy greens, such as kale, spinach, and/or a spring mix

$^1/_2$ cucumber, cut into chunks

1 celery stalk, cut into chunks

1 tablespoon lemon juice

1 teaspoon honey, agave syrup, or equivalent sweetener
such as stevia, if desired

1 cup Thick-Style Coconut Milk (page 142),
Thin-Style Coconut Milk (page 142),
or cow's or goat's milk while gradually increasing
your coconut oil intake

2 tablespoons vanilla flavored or unflavored
whey protein powder

Extra coconut oil (melted) or MCT and
Coconut Oil 4:3 Mixture (page 141) (optional)

Directions: Place all the ingredients in a blender, add the coconut oil or the MCT and coconut oil mixture if using, and process for about 30 seconds until smooth and creamy. If mixture is too thick, add more coconut milk as needed.

MARY'S FAVORITE GREEK YOGURT BREAKFAST

YIELD: One serving

. . . .

$1/2$ cup plain full-fat Greek yogurt

8 drops liquid stevia (or 1 to 2 teaspoons honey)

1 tablespoon unsweetened grated coconut

$1/4$ cup mixed unsalted organic nuts
(walnuts, pecans, cashews, almonds and Brazil nuts)

4 ounces coconut milk for drinking

Directions: Place the yogurt into a breakfast bowl. Mix the stevia or honey into the yogurt thoroughly with a spoon. Sprinkle the coconut and nuts on top, and mix in. Enjoy with a glass of coconut milk on the side.

MARY'S RICOTTA CONCOCTION (BREAKFAST OR SNACK)

YIELD: One serving

. . . .

$1/2$ cup full-fat ricotta cheese

8 to 10 drops stevia

2 ounces coconut milk

$1/4$ cup sliced almonds or chopped walnuts

1 tablespoon unsweetened grated coconut

Directions: Place the ricotta into a small dish. Mix the stevia and coconut milk into the ricotta thoroughly with a spoon, then add the nuts and grated coconut and stir again.

TASTY COTTAGE CHEESE AND OIL MIX

YIELD: One serving

• •

4 ounces cottage cheese

Your usual serving of MCT oil or MCT and
Coconut Oil 4:3 Mixture (page 141)

Directions: Place the cottage cheese and the coconut oil or MCT/coconut oil mixture into a small dish. Mix together with a fork or spoon.

CHEESY SCRAMBLED EGGS

YIELD: Two eggs

• •

1 tablespoon coconut oil

2 eggs

2 tablespoons coconut milk

Pinch of sea salt

2 tablespoons grated or shredded cheese

Directions: Melt the coconut oil in a skillet on low-medium heat. Break the eggs into a small bowl and scramble them and the coconut milk vigorously with a fork or wire whisk. Whisk in the salt and cheese and pour into the heated skillet. Use a spatula to scrape the cooked egg off the bottom of the skillet, turning the egg over repeatedly until the egg is no longer liquid but still fluffy and moist.

Variations: Whisk some chopped parsley, spinach, green pepper, or green onions into the mixture before adding to the skillet.

WHATEVER FRITTATA

YIELD: Four servings

• •

3 tablespoons coconut oil

About 2 cups fresh vegetables or
1 bag defrosted frozen vegetables of your choice

Salt and pepper

Sprinkling of a favorite spice mix (optional)

$3/4$ cup shredded cheese of your choice
or $1/2$ cup crumbled feta cheese

6 eggs

1 tablespoon grated Parmesan
or Romano cheese

Directions: Select an omelet-style skillet that can also be used in the oven. Place the oven rack about 5 inches below the broiler and preheat it to a high temperature. Crack the eggs into a medium-size bowl. Warm the coconut oil in the skillet on low-medium heat. Add the vegetables and sauté the vegetables in the oil, stirring often, until tender, about 4 to 5 minutes.

While the vegetables are cooking, beat the eggs with a wire whisk, add the cheese and several pinches of salt, and mix thoroughly.

When the vegetables are nearly finished, season with salt and pepper and spice mix if using. Stir well and distribute the vegetables evenly around the bottom of the skillet.

When the vegetables are ready, pour the egg mixture evenly over them and continue to cook undisturbed for about 4 to 5 minutes until the edges of the frittata are dry and slightly brown; the egg mixture will appear runny on the top.

Sprinkle the Parmesan or Romano cheese evenly on top of the frittata and place it under the broiler for at least 3 minutes. Be sure to set a timer to avoid burning it.

After 3 minutes, open the oven and pull the rack out just enough to check the frittata. With an oven glove on your hand, shake the handle of the skillet gently; if the top does not jiggle and appears lightly browned, the frittata is set and ready to be removed from the oven. If the top jiggles, replace it under broiler for 1 to 2 more minutes, watch closely, then check again. Allow the frittata to cool for at least 5 minutes, then cut it into quarters and serve.

Variation: Add 1 to 2 cups of leftover chopped meat, fish, or poultry of any kind. You can add whatever you like!

SPINACH AND FETA OMELET

YIELD: One serving

4 teaspoons coconut oil

1 cup fresh spinach leaves

2 or 3 eggs

2 tablespoons coconut milk

Pinch of sea salt for each egg

Pepper to taste

2 ounces crumbled feta cheese, about $1/2$ cup

Directions: Warm 2 teaspoons of the coconut oil in a nonstick omelet-style skillet on low-medium heat. Add the spinach and sauté until just wilted; remove it from the pan and set aside.

With a wire whisk beat the eggs, then whisk in the coconut milk, salt, and pepper. Add 2 more teaspoons of coconut oil to the skillet and when heated, pour the egg evenly into the hot skillet. Leave it undisturbed for several minutes.

When the omelet is set on the edges with some wet egg still on top, carefully flip the omelet with a spatula. Evenly distribute the spinach and feta over half the omelet and use the spatula to fold the omelet in half covering the spinach and cheese. When the cheese inside begins to melt, the omelet is done.

MARGARITA FRITTATA

YIELD: Four servings

· ·

4 tablespoons coconut oil

1 tablespoon minced garlic

2 cups fresh spinach leaves

Salt and pepper

6 to 8 eggs

$1/_2$ teaspoon basil, dry or fresh, minced

8 cherry tomatoes, halved

4 ounces fresh mozzarella ball, cut into four slices

Directions: Select an omelet-style skillet that can also be used in the oven. Place the oven rack about 5 inches below the broiler and preheat it to a high temperature. Crack the eggs into a medium-size bowl.

Warm the coconut oil in the skillet on low-medium heat. Sauté the minced garlic in the oil for a few seconds, then add the spinach, stirring often, until almost wilted, about 1 to 2 minutes. Sprinkle the spinach lightly with salt when nearly finished and mix well. Distribute the spinach evenly around the bottom of the skillet.

While the spinach is cooking, beat the eggs with a wire whisk. Add a pinch of salt for every two eggs, and whisk again thoroughly.

When the spinach is ready, pour the egg mixture evenly over the spinach and immediately use a heat-resistant spoon or spatula to swirl the spinach into egg mixture. Drop the cherry tomato halves evenly into the frittata. Continue to cook the frittata undisturbed for about 4 to 5 minutes until the edges are dry and slightly brown; the egg mixture will appear runny on the top. Just before removing from the stovetop, place one mozzarella slice flat on top of each quarter of the frittata. Remove from the skillet and place it under broiler for at least three minutes. Be sure to set a timer to avoid burning.

After three minutes, open the oven and pull the rack out just enough to check the frittata. With an oven glove on your hand, shake the handle of the skillet gently; if the egg portion does not jiggle and appear lightly browned, the frittata is set and ready to be removed from the oven. The now-melted mozzarella might move with this maneuver. If the top jiggles, replace it under broiler for 1 to 2 more minutes and check again. Allow the frittata to cool for at least five minutes, then cut it into quarters and serve.

MARY'S FAVORITE OMELET

YIELD: One serving

1 tablespoon coconut oil

2 or 3 eggs

2 tablespoons coconut milk

2 pinches of salt

Pepper to taste

4 cherry tomatoes, halved

6 Kalamata olives, halved and pitted

$1^1/_2$ ounces shredded cheddar cheese, about $^1/_3$ cup

Directions: Warm the coconut oil in a nonstick omelet-style skillet over low-medium heat. With a wire whisk, beat the eggs, then whisk in the coconut milk and the salt and pepper, and pour evenly into the hot skillet. Leave the egg undisturbed for several minutes.

When the omelet is about set on the edges with some wet egg still on top, carefully flip the omelet with a spatula. Evenly distribute the tomato and olive pieces as well as about 1 ounce of the cheese on half of the omelet, and use the spatula to fold the omelet in half covering the vegetables and cheese. Distribute the rest of the cheese evenly over the top of the folded omelet. When the cheese on the top begins to melt, the omelet is done.

Variations: Make a Greek-style omelet by using two to three large spoonfuls of Greek Salad (page 156) and feta cheese in place of the other vegetables and cheese.

SOUP AND SANDWICH

GRILLED CHEESE SANDWICH

YIELD: One sandwich
(about 2 tablespoons of coconut oil)

• •

2 slices whole-grain or gluten-free bread

2 to 3 ounces favorite sliced cheese

2 tablespoons coconut oil

Directions: Place the cheese between the two slices of bread and spread one tablespoon of coconut oil on the outer surface of both sides of the sandwich. Cook over low-medium heat on each side until lightly browned and the cheese is beginning to melt.

Variation: Place a layer of thinly sliced tomatoes and/or spinach on top of the cheese.

MANY COLORS VEGETABLE SOUP

YIELD: About six to twelve servings

• •

3 tablespoons coconut oil

2 tablespoons minced garlic

1 cup broccoli florets

1 cup cauliflower florets

1 large tomato, chopped

$1/2$ to 1 cup chopped yellow sweet or bell peppers

1 cup chopped or shredded carrot

1 cup chopped celery

1 cup chopped mushrooms

$1/2$ large red or sweet onion, chopped

2 teaspoons sea salt (or more to taste)

$1/4$ teaspoon white or black pepper (or more to taste)

6 to 9 cups vegetable broth or chicken or beef stock

For each serving: Your usual serving of coconut oil, MCT oil,
or MCT and Coconut Oil 4:3 Mixture (page 141)

Directions: Set a soup pot on the stove over medium-low heat. Add 3 table-spoons of coconut oil and sauté the minced garlic for a few seconds. Add the vegetables and continue to sauté until all the vegetables are tender, about 10 minutes.

Add the broth or stock to the soup pot and simmer over low heat for about one hour. When ready to serve, drizzle each bowl with your usual serving of coconut oil, MCT oil, or MCT/coconut oil mixture. Store the remaining soup in the refrigerator.

Variation: Add 1 or 2 cups of tomato sauce in place of an equal amount of broth or stock.

SALADS AND SAUCES

CHOPPED GREEK SALAD

YIELD: Six to eight servings

. . . .

1 15-ounce can of garbanzo beans, drained
(for lower carb salad, use 8-ounce can)

1 large cucumber, chopped

1 large bell pepper, chopped

$1/2$ large sweet onion, chopped

1 medium tomato, chopped

25 to 30 Kalamata or black olives, pitted

1 to 2 ounces of crumbled feta or goat cheese per serving,
about $1/4$ to $1/2$ cup, as desired

About 6 cups leafy green and purple spring mix

Salad dressing:

3 tablespoons olive oil

$1^1/2$ tablespoons lemon juice

$1/4$ teaspoon sea salt

2 teaspoons Greek seasoning
(salt, garlic powder, black pepper, oregano, sage)

Additional salad dressing, per serving:

Your usual serving MCT oil or MCT and Coconut Oil 4:3 Mixture
(page 141)

Directions: To a large bowl or storage container, add the garbanzo beans, chopped cucumber, bell pepper, onion, and tomato, and toss together with all the salad dressing ingredients except for the MCT oil or coconut/MCT oil mixture. This can be stored in the refrigerator for two to three days.

When ready to serve, add a serving of the leafy spring mix to medium-size salad bowls, about half filled. Add two to three large serving spoonfuls of the dressed vegetable mixture. Evenly distribute crumbled cheese over the vegetables and top with four to five olives. Now pour the MCT oil or MCT/coconut oil mixture evenly over the salad and toss.

Variation: At the time of serving, add fresh cooked or canned beets (not pickled), chopped. If added beforehand, the beets will discolor the other vegetables.

Chicken Salad

YIELD: Two to four servings

. . . .

2 cups chopped, cooked chicken

$1/_2$ cup chopped celery

$1/_2$ cup sliced almonds or chopped walnuts

$1/_4$ cup mayonnaise

2 tablespoons MCT oil or MCT/
Coconut Oil 4:3 Mixture (page 141)

Salt and pepper to taste

Directions: Toss the chicken, celery, and nuts together in a medium-size bowl. In a separate bowl, use a wire whisk to thoroughly blend the mayonnaise and the MCT oil or MCT/coconut oil mixture, and then add it the to chicken mixture. Season to taste with salt and pepper and toss again until well mixed.

Optional: Mix additional MCT oil or MCT/coconut oil mixture into your serving.

Variations: Add one of the following: $1/_4$ cup raisins, 16 grapes cut in half, or 8 pitted Kalamata or black olives cut in half.

TUNA SALAD

YIELD: About two servings

• •

2 5-ounce cans of tuna, drained

$1/4$ cup chopped sweet onion

2 tablespoons sweet pickle relish or dill pickle relish
(a lower carb choice)

2 tablespoons mayonnaise

1 tablespoon MCT oil or MCT and Coconut Oil 4:3 Mixture (page 141)

Salt and pepper to taste

Directions: Toss the tuna, onion, and relish together in a medium-size bowl. In a separate bowl, use a wire whisk to thoroughly blend the mayonnaise and the MCT oil or MCT/coconut oil mixture, and then add it to the tuna mixture. Season to taste with salt and pepper and toss again until well mixed.

Optional: Mix additional MCT oil or MCT/coconut oil mixture into your serving.

CALIFORNIA SALAD

YIELD: One serving

• •

2 cups mixed colors of salad greens

10 to 12 pieces dried cherries

2 heaping tablespoons chopped walnuts

1 ounce Gorgonzola cheese, about $1/4$ cup, broken apart

Salad dressing:

1 tablespoon MCT and Coconut Oil 4:3 Mixture (page 141)

$1/2$ tablespoon walnut oil

$1/4$ to $1/2$ teaspoon raspberry balsamic vinegar (to taste)

Directions: Place the salad greens in a medium-size salad bowl. Sprinkle the cherries, walnuts, and cheese on top of the greens. Mix the dressing ingredients in a small bowl, then pour evenly over the salad and toss before serving.

MANY COLORS SALAD

YIELD: About 6 servings

• •

1 cup broccoli florets

1 cup cauliflower florets

1 cup halved red cherry tomatoes

$1/2$ to 1 cup chopped yellow sweet or bell pepper

2 carrots, chopped

1 cup chopped mushrooms

$1/2$ large sweet or purple onion, chopped

About 6 cups leafy green and purple spring mix

$1^1/2$ cups shredded cheddar cheese

Salad dressing:

6 tablespoons of your favorite salad dressing

6 tablespoons MCT oil or MCT and
Coconut Oil 4:3 Mixture (page 141)

Directions: Wash the vegetables and the spring mix thoroughly. When dry, place the ingredients in a large salad bowl with the cheese and toss together.

Place the ingredients for the salad dressing in a small bowl and mix with a wire whisk. Pour immediately onto the salad and toss again just before serving.

Variation: Toss all the vegetables together, except for the spring mix, and use for two or three days by storing in refrigerator. When time to serve, add about 1 cup of the vegetable mix to 1 cup of the spring mix and toss with 2 tablespoons of Simple Salad Dressing or Vegetable Topping (page 160).

SIMPLE SALAD DRESSING OR VEGETABLE TOPPING

YIELD: One or two servings

• •

1 tablespoon of your favorite salad dressing

1 tablespoon MCT oil or MCT and Coconut Oil 4:3 Mixture (page 141)

Directions: Place the ingredients in a small bowl. Mix together with a wire whisk and pour immediately onto salad greens or vegetables, and toss. Excess dressing can be stored in the refrigerator, and then rewarmed and remixed before serving.

SIMPLE TOPPING FOR CHICKEN OR CHICKEN SALAD

YIELD: One serving

• •

1 tablespoon of honey-Dijon or ranch-style salad dressing

1 tablespoon MCT oil or MCT and Coconut Oil 4:3 Mixture (page 141)

Directions: Mix the ingredients together with a wire whisk and pour immediately onto the chicken or mix into the chicken salad.

SIMPLE TARTAR SAUCE

YIELD: A half cup

• •

4 tablespoons mayonnaise

2 tablespoons MCT oil or MCT and Coconut Oil 4:3 Mixture (page 141)

1 teaspoon lemon juice

1 teaspoon prepared yellow mustard

1 tablespoon sweet pickle relish or dill pickle relish (a lower carb choice)

Directions: In a small bowl, use a wire whisk to blend the mayonnaise and the MCT oil or MCT/coconut oil mixture. Blend in the lemon juice and yellow mustard, then add the relish and mix again.

ENTICING ENTREES

SYBIL'S COCONUT CHICKEN TENDERS OR FISH FINGERS

YIELD: Four servings

· ·

1 whole egg, beaten

$1/2$ cup whole-wheat panko or Italian bread crumbs

$1/2$ cup unsweetened grated coconut

$1/4$ cup grated Parmesan cheese

1 teaspoon garlic salt

$1/4$ teaspoon pepper

3 tablespoons coconut oil

1 tablespoon olive or canola oil

12 fresh raw chicken tenders or cod fish filets, cut into strips

Directions: Beat the egg with a fork in a bowl. Combine all the dry ingredients on a large plate and mix thoroughly with a fork. Place the chicken tenders or fish fingers in the bowl with the egg and stir until all are thoroughly coated.

Meanwhile, heat the coconut oil and the olive or canola oil in a large skillet over medium heat.

Roll each tender in the dry mix until it is covered and set aside on another plate. When all the chicken tenders or fish fingers are coated, place them in the hot oil in the skillet and cook for about 3 to 4 minutes on each side until done.

Variation: Serve the chicken with Simple Topping for Chicken (page 160) and the fish fingers with Simple Tartar Sauce (page 160).

STIR-FRIED NAPA CABBAGE WITH CARROTS AND COCONUT

YIELD: 4 servings

2$^{1}/_{2}$ tablespoons teriyaki sauce

1 teaspoon sesame oil

$^{1}/_{4}$ teaspoon salt

$^{1}/_{8}$ teaspoon pepper

2 tablespoons coconut oil

1 tablespoon peanut oil

1 heaping tablespoon minced garlic

1 tablespoon minced, peeled, fresh ginger

2 cups shredded carrots

$^{1}/_{2}$ cup flaked coconut

1 medium Napa (also called Chinese) cabbage, thinly sliced

Minced cilantro or parsley to taste

Salt and pepper to taste

Directions: Put the teriyaki sauce, sesame oil, and salt and pepper in a small bowl. Combine well and set aside.

In a wok or large skillet, warm the coconut and peanut oils over medium-high heat. When hot, add the garlic and ginger and stir for several seconds. Add the carrots and flaked coconut and stir-fry for about 3 minutes. Add the sliced cabbage and stir-fry for about 3 more minutes until tender. Add the teriyaki mixture and toss with the vegetable mixture until thoroughly coated.

Remove the vegetables from the heat to avoid overcooking. Sprinkle with the parsley or cilantro and season with salt and pepper. Toss again and serve immediately.

Variation: After the vegetables and teriyaki mixture are combined, stir in the cooked Stir-Fried Chicken Tenders (page 163) and warm together for 1 minute.

CASHEW CHICKEN

YIELD: Four servings

• • • • • • • • • • • • • • • • • • • •

2$^1/_2$ tablespoons teriyaki sauce

1 teaspoon sesame oil

$^1/_4$ teaspoon salt

$^1/_8$ teaspoon pepper

12 Stir-Fried Chicken Tenders (below), cooked

$^1/_2$ cup cashews

2 cups fresh broccoli florets, cut into small pieces

Salt and pepper to taste

Directions: Put the teriyaki sauce, sesame oil, and salt and pepper in a small bowl. Combine well and set aside. When the chicken tenders are thoroughly cooked, turn down the heat to low. Add the teriyaki sauce, cashews, and broccoli florets, and stir constantly for 1 or 2 more minutes. Season to taste with salt and pepper.

STIR-FRIED CHICKEN TENDERS

YIELD: Four servings

• • • • • • • • • • • • • • • • • • • •

4 tablespoons coconut oil

1 tablespoon peanut or sesame oil,
plus 2 teaspoons sesame oil

2 teaspoons cornstarch

1 tablespoon minced garlic

1 teaspoon minced, peeled, fresh ginger

12 fresh raw chicken tenders

Directions: Warm the coconut oil and 1 tablespoon of the peanut or sesame oil in a large wok or skillet on the stove over medium heat.

Meanwhile, in a large bowl, make a paste with the cornstarch and 2 teaspoons of the sesame oil. Add the chicken tenders and gently mix until completely coated with the paste.

When the oil in the skillet is hot, add the garlic and ginger and stir briefly, then add the tenders and cook for 3 to 4 minutes on each side until thoroughly cooked.

SIMPLE SALMON DINNER

YIELD: Two servings

• •

2 whole sweet potatoes or yams

Olive oil spray

10 to 12 ounces salmon fillet, any size

1 bunch fresh asparagus

2 to 3 tablespoons coconut oil, melted

Finely chopped garlic or garlic powder and dried herb,
such as dill or thyme, or other favorite seasoning

Additional $1/2$ to 1 tablespoon coconut oil per sweet potato or yam

Directions: Preheat the oven to 350°F. Wash, dry, and pierce the sweet potatoes several times with a fork and place them on the oven rack to cook for 25 to 30 minutes.

Place aluminum foil on a large cookie sheet or spray the cookie sheet with olive oil spray. On one side of the cookie sheet place the salmon fillet, skin side down, and on the other evenly distribute the asparagus spears. Melt 2 to 3 tablespoons of coconut oil (or more for a very large fillet), and coat the salmon and asparagus with the oil using a pastry brush. Sprinkle the garlic and herb or other seasoning over the fish and asparagus.

When the sweet potatoes have been in the oven for 25 to 30 minutes, move them to the side and place the cookie sheet with the fish and asparagus in the oven. Bake for 20 minutes longer. The salmon should be very moist and separate easily with a fork. Open each sweet potato, cut grooves with a knife, and spoon $1/2$ to 1 tablespoon of coconut oil onto each potato.

STUFFED BELL PEPPERS

YIELD: Five servings

· ·

2 tablespoons olive oil

5 large bell peppers of various colors

3 tablespoons coconut oil

1 large sweet onion, chopped

7 cloves garlic, minced

1 pound ground beef or ground turkey

2 cups tomato sauce

3 cups chicken broth

$3/4$ cup uncooked whole-grain rice

$1/2$ teaspoon sea salt

$1/4$ teaspoon black pepper

1 tablespoon dried peppermint, plus an additional 1 teaspoon

Directions: Preheat the oven to 300°F. Cut the tops off the peppers, then split the peppers in half lengthwise. Spread the olive oil on the bottom of a 9-by-12-inch baking pan and lay the peppers on it open side up. Bake in the oven for about 40 minutes while preparing the remaining ingredients. Remove the stems from the pepper tops and chop the remaining pepper pieces.

In a large skillet, heat the coconut oil over medium-low heat and sauté the garlic, onion, and pepper pieces until tender. Add the ground beef or turkey and use a fork to break apart; stir until thoroughly cooked. Add 1 cup of the tomato sauce (reserve the other cup for later), 2 cups of the broth, and the rice. Cover with a lid and simmer over low heat for 30 minutes, stirring occasionally. Add the salt and pepper, and 1 tablespoon of peppermint and stir thoroughly.

Remove the peppers from the oven and increase the temperature to 375°F. Fill the roasted pepper halves with equal amounts of meat mixture. Spoon 1 cup of tomato sauce over the tops of the meat mixture, then sprinkle lightly with salt, pepper, and the remaining peppermint. Form a tent with aluminum foil over the top of the baking pan so that foil does not stick to tomato topping. Return the pan to the oven and bake for 40 minutes.

VEGETABLE SIDE DISHES

Brussels Sprouts

YIELD: Three to four servings

· ·

2 tablespoons coconut oil

1 pound of small Brussels sprouts

1/2 teaspoon garlic salt with parsley

Directions: Using your favorite steaming method, steam the Brussels sprouts for 4 to 5 minutes or until tender. Place the hot Brussels sprouts in a bowl, add the coconut oil, and sprinkle the garlic salt evenly over the sprouts. Toss until all the ingredients are evenly distributed.

Garlicky Spinach

YIELD: Two to three servings

· ·

2 tablespoons coconut oil

1 level tablespoon minced garlic

1 bunch fresh spinach

1/4 teaspoon sea salt

Directions: Warm the coconut oil in a large skillet just below medium heat. When heated, add the minced garlic and use a spatula to distribute over the surface. Add the spinach and stir with the spatula until all the leaves are moist and slightly wilted but not soggy. Sprinkle the spinach with sea salt, stir in quickly, and then remove from the skillet to avoid overcooking.

Variations: Add a heaping tablespoon of pine nuts along with the garlic.

ALMOND BROCCOLI

YIELD: Two to three servings

• •

1 bunch broccoli, cut into bite-size pieces

2 tablespoons coconut oil

$1/4$ teaspoon sea salt

$1/4$ cup sliced almonds

Directions: Using your favorite steaming method, steam the broccoli for 4 to 5 minutes. Place the hot broccoli in a bowl, add the coconut oil, and sprinkle the salt evenly over the mixture. Then add the sliced almonds and toss the ingredients until evenly distributed.

Variation: Use cauliflower instead of broccoli.

SAUTÉED GREENS WITH GARLIC

YIELD: Two to three servings

• •

1 bunch kale, red or green chard, or beet greens

2 tablespoons coconut oil

I garlic clove, minced or thinly sliced

Juice of $1/2$ lemon

Salt to taste

Directions: Rinse the greens and remove the stems from leaves. Cut the stems into $1/2$-inch segments and set aside. Chop the leaves into small pieces.

Heat the coconut oil in a large skillet over medium-low heat and add the garlic, sautéing until it starts to change color. Add the stems and stir occasionally for about 2 minutes until almost tender. Add the chopped leaves, partially covering skillet with the lid, and continue to cook for 3 to 5 more minutes. Add the lemon juice and salt to taste, and then toss until thoroughly distributed. Remove the greens from the skillet and serve.

CREAMY DELIGHTS

Coconut Macaroons

YIELD: Eighteen small cookies

. . . .

2 egg whites

Pinch of salt

$1/_2$ teaspoon vanilla, chocolate,
or almond extract

$2/_3$ cup sugar

1 cup shredded coconut

Directions: Preheat the oven to 325°F. Beat the egg whites with the salt and extract until soft peaks form. Gradually add the sugar and beat until stiff. Fold in the coconut.

Grease a cookie sheet with a generous amount of butter. Drop the batter by the rounded teaspoon onto the cookie sheet. Bake for 20 minutes. Each cookie contains approximately 4 grams (almost 1 teaspoon) of coconut oil.

Variation: Instead of $2/_3$ cup of sugar, add 1 to 2 dashes of liquid stevia extract or equivalent granulated sweetener to $1/_4$ cup of sugar.

Coconut-Chocolate Dip or Topping

YIELD: About 16 ounces

. . . .

1 cup coconut oil

1 cup (8 ounces) dark or milk chocolate chips or squares
(if chocolate is unsweetened, add 3 tablespoons
or more of honey to taste)

Directions: Melt the coconut oil in a small saucepan over very low heat. Add the chocolate and stir continuously until thoroughly blended. Serve immediately as a topping for ice cream or as a dip for strawberries or other fruits or nuts.

Variations: For chocolate-covered fruits or nuts, dip each piece into the chocolate, then place it on a plate with the others and refrigerate for eating later.

COCONUT FUDGE OR CANDIES

YIELD: About 16 ounces

• •

1 cup coconut oil

1 cup (8 ounces) dark or milk chocolate chips or squares
(if chocolate is unsweetened, add 3 tablespoons
or more of honey to taste)

Directions: Melt the coconut oil in a small saucepan over very low heat. Add the chocolate and stir continuously until thoroughly blended.

Divide the mixture equally into paper candy cups on a large plate or into a plastic ice cube tray.

Place in the freezer and chill until set. In a sixteen-cube tray, each cube will equal 1 tablespoon of coconut oil and will easily pop out of the tray. Store the candy in the refrigerator or freezer.

Variations: Add $1/4$ cup of grated coconut and/or chopped nuts to part or all of the oil and chocolate mixture. Or put some of the mixture in the bottom of the candy cups or sections of the ice cube tray, add a dollop of peanut butter or several pieces of creamed coconut and then top each candy piece with remainder of the mixture.

## PART TWO

Disorders That May Respond to Ketones

with Caregiver Reports and Personal Accounts

6

An Analysis of Caregiver Reports for People with Dementias and Other Memory Impairment

I have received e-mails and letters from more than 400 people who have communicated results of using coconut oil, MCT oil, or both, mostly on behalf of their loved ones and occasionally for themselves. I have taken their reports and attempted to organize the improvements into categories. I do not consider this a scientific trial by any means, and I believe that people are more likely to write to me if they have experienced improvement than if they have not. I do not prompt them with regard to what type of improvements to expect; if they do not provide details, I simply ask them to write to me again to give me the details of what they are observing. I also ask people who inquire about using coconut oil or MCT oil to let me know how the person responds, even if they do not. Even though this is not a clinical trial, improvement in such a large number of people suggests that there is something to this dietary strategy and that clinical trials are warranted.

TYPES OF IMPROVEMENTS

In the reports sent to me from caregivers of the people with a diagnosis of dementia or some other type of memory impairment,

91 percent feel they have seen some type of improvement. Another 3 percent say that they did not see a specific improvement, however, they also did not see a worsening of symptoms over a period of six months or longer. And 6 percent did not notice any improvement or stabilization.

Approximately, 60 percent reported some improvement in memory and/or cognition in their loved ones; 40 percent an improvement in their mood, behavior, or interaction with other people; and 35 percent report an improvement in their language and/or conversational skills, including several who had stopped talking and resumed talking. In one case, a wife reported that her husband, who had not spoken in more than a year, resumed speaking in lengthy, grammatically correct sentences shortly after starting coconut oil. Approximately, one in four people reported that they resumed activities that they had been unable to perform or had not performed for a period of time, ranging from carrying out their own personal hygiene unassisted to playing with grandchildren, reading, writing, knitting, sewing, completing crossword puzzles, and performing housework or yard work. Approximately, one in five reported improvement in their physical symptoms, such as having fewer tremors or being better able to get up and walk around, and for a few there was improved sleep, appetite, or vision. Many people experienced improvement in several categories.

While many people report some type of measurable memory or cognitive improvement, there are also quality-of-life improvements that cannot easily be measured. Renewed recognition of loved ones and return of one's personality and sense of humor might not be quantifiable, but the benefit to oneself and one's loved ones is immeasurable.

For the conference Dietary Therapies for Epilepsy and Other Neurological Disorders held in Chicago in 2012, I prepared a poster presentation that included a chart of the types of responses to coconut oil, MCT oil, or both in people with dementia and memory impairment reported to me by caregivers. These responses, compiled below, include the verbatim phrases used in these reports that helped me categorize the kinds of improvements people are seeing.

Improved Memory/Cognition

- Able to do mental math again
- Higher scores on memory or cognitive test
- More awareness of time and place
- Recognizing people or places
- Improved reading comprehension

- Improved clock drawing
- Better sense of direction
- More alert
- Brighter
- Improved awareness
- Less foggy
- Less hazy
- Less distractible
- Better cognition

Improved Social Interaction, Behavior, Mood

- More interaction with others
- Better sense of humor
- Less agitation
- Improved behavior
- Less hostile

- Less aggressive
- Happy
- Improved mood
- Less anxiety
- Less depression
- Feels better

Improved Speech, Conversation

- Improved conversation
- More talkative
- Improved verbal skills
- Better word recall
- Expressing thoughts

- Speaking again
- Clearer speech
- Less repetitiveness
- Making sense
- More logical

Resumption of Lost Activities

- Showering again without help
- Performing self-care again
- Doing things around the house
- Doing household chores again
- Preparing meals again
- More functional
- Resumed a hobby
- Reading again

Improved Physical Symptoms

- Fewer episodes of faintness, clamminess, sweating
- Getting out of bed without help
- Fewer episodes of seizure/twitching
- Able to walk again
- Walking without assistance
- Improved strength
- More ambulatory
- More energy
- Less stiffness
- Improved balance
- Less dizziness
- Less tremor
- Improved gait
- Pain relief

Improved Sleep

- No longer twitching during sleep
- No longer sleeping excessively
- Fewer nightmares
- Sleeping better

Improved Vision

- Visual disturbance gone
- Able to see more clearly

Improved Appetite

Table 6.1 presents the percentage of people who showed improvement within each of these categories.

TABLE 6.1. IMPROVEMENTS OBSERVED AFTER CONSUMING MEDIUM-CHAIN FATTY ACIDS		
OVERALL RESPONSE	**NUMBER AFFECTED**	**PERCENT AFFECTED**
Improved	167/184	91
Improved memory/cognition	108/184	59
Did not improve	11/184	6
Stable over 6 months	5/184	3
SPECIFIC RESPONSES		
Improved social/behavior/mood	77/184	42
Improved speech/verbal skills	64/184	35
Resumption of lost activities	44/184	24
Improved physical symptoms	38/184	21
Improvement, otherwise unspecified	10/184	5
Improved sleep	8/184	4
Improved appetite	6/184	3
Improved vision	2/184	1

Figure 6.1 (page 178) presents a chart of people who showed improvement within each of these categories.

PATIENCE AND PERSISTENCE MAY PAY OFF

Of the hundreds of people who have tried this approach and reported back to me, I have heard every variation of response from no response at all after several months of trying to some obvious improvement after the very first dose. While some people seem to have an immediate response to coconut or MCT oil even at smaller amounts (one or two teaspoons), most people see improvements more gradually using larger amounts, or they see stabilization that

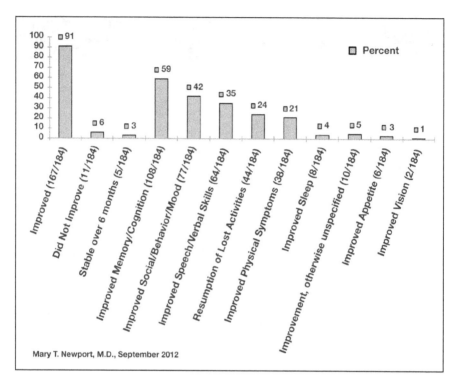

Figure 6.1. Responses of People with Dementia and Other Memory
Impairment to Medium-Chain Fatty Acids (N=184)

becomes more obvious when symptoms have not worsened notice-
ably over several months. Therefore, try not to be discouraged if
you don't see immediate and dramatic results. It is not known at
this time why some people have a dramatic response to ketones and
others do not. High-insulin levels can inhibit ketone production, so
it is quite conceivable that an excessive intake of carbohydrates in
the diet, which raises insulin levels, could be a factor for some people. Also, it is likely that a genetic component plays a role in certain
people. Hopefully, clinical trials now in progress will provide an
answer.

7

Alzheimer's Disease

The rate of Alzheimer's disease, like obesity and type 2 diabetes, has risen to epidemic proportions worldwide over the past several decades. According to the *2014 Facts and Figures* report from the Alzheimer's Association, available from their website at www.alz.org, an estimated 5.2 million Americans are believed to currently suffer with this degenerative brain disease, with roughly half undiagnosed, and about 200,000 under the age of sixty-five with the "early-onset" form of the disease. The number of people with Alzheimer's disease nearly doubles for each five-year interval over age sixty-five, such that people who live beyond eighty-five years of age have a 32 percent chance of developing the disease. As the generation of baby boomers reaches their mid-sixties and beyond, unless a medical breakthrough identifies ways to prevent or treat the disease, by 2050, the number of Alzheimer's victims is predicted to triple to a staggering 13.8 million people in the United States alone, and to more than 100 million worldwide.

These figures leveled off between 2013 and 2014 and are down somewhat compared to the organization's *2012 Facts and Figures* report. In the summer of 2013, results of three new studies were published showing that rates of dementia are actually declining in England, Sweden, and the Netherlands; for example, people born later in the twentieth century in England have a lower risk of dementia at the same age than people born earlier. A myriad of factors could account for the difference in those countries, including those related to diet, tobacco smoking, and improvements in medical care, just to mention a few.

More women than men develop the disease, but this is attributed for the most part to the greater lifespan of women. People who are Hispanic or African-American and age eighty-five or older are roughly twice as likely to develop Alzheimer's disease compared to Caucasian Americans. Other health factors, such as higher rates of diabetes and high blood pressure in certain ethnic groups, appear to explain the difference.

According to the Alzheimer's Association, Alzheimer's disease is currently the sixth leading cause of death in the United States overall, and the fifth leading cause for people over age sixty-five. These figures are based on information from death certificates. But a 2014 report in the journal *Neurology* states that a more accurate estimate, based on autopsy data, would increase the actual number of Alzheimer's deaths from just under 84,000 in 2010 to more than 503,000, bringing it to third place for cause of death—not far behind the higher ranked heart disease at 598,000 and cancer at 575,000 (James, 2014). People with Alzheimer's disease often die as a direct result of their disease, such as the inability to eat or the aspiration of food due to poor swallowing, which can result in pneumonia, but the death certificate may not reflect Alzheimer's as the underlying cause of these serious problems.

The National Center for Health Statistics reported that, while death rates from stroke, heart disease, and certain cancers declined between 2000 and 2006, deaths from Alzheimer's disease increased by 47.1 percent.

The annual costs of caring for people with Alzheimer's disease to U.S. government and businesses is currently estimated at an astounding $203 billion, with the lion's share, 70 percent, paid by Medicare and Medicaid; 17 percent paid out-of-pocket by the patient and family; and only 13 percent paid by private insurers, HMOs, and managed care plans. In addition, the Alzheimer's Association estimates that 17.7 billion hours of unpaid caregiving are provided annually for people with Alzheimer's and other dementias, equivalent to about $220.2 billion if such care was provided by paid attendants at the rate of $12.45 per hour.

ALZHEIMER'S DISEASE: THE MOST COMMON FORM OF DEMENTIA

Alzheimer's disease is a progressive brain disease that is considered to be irreversible. It is a mysterious process that causes brain cells to lose their connections with one another and subsequently die. In spite of intense worldwide research since the early 1970s, the exact cause that sets off the cascade of events in this disease and other related dementias is still unknown in 2014.

When someone younger than sixty-five develops this type of dementia, it is called "early-onset" Alzheimer's disease. An estimated 200,000 people, about 3.8 percent of the 5.2 million affected in the United States, fall into this category. Alzheimer's disease has even been described in people in their thirties and forties, particularly those with the familial form of the disease, which represents only 0.1 percent of the total number of cases. People sixty-five and older are considered to have "late-onset" Alzheimer's disease and represent the vast majority of cases.

Recent advances in imaging technologies have made it possible to detect subtle changes in the brain a decade or more before a person develops obvious symptoms of the disease. The amyloid-PET scan can give us an idea of how much plaque is present in the brain and where it is concentrated. However, this method is not perfect; people with a diagnosis of Alzheimer's disease, based on testing and symptoms, may have relatively little plaque, and some people of advanced age with no signs of the disease may have large areas of plaque. As these techniques are improved and other tests are developed, such advances will make it possible for people who are at risk to become more proactive on their own behalf. Preventive measures such as quitting smoking, controlling blood pressure, increasing exercise, treating sleep apnea, adopting a healthier diet, and staying mentally active can protect against and reverse the effects of impaired insulin-related conditions. While the cause or causes of Alzheimer's are not known, such lifestyle changes, particularly if adopted sooner rather than later, could potentially prevent, delay the onset, or otherwise alter the course of the disease.

DNA testing, which can be accomplished with a blood test or even by submitting saliva, can give us an idea of risk based on whether we have inherited ApoE4 genes from our parents, which places a person at greater than average, but not at definite risk, compared to someone who carries ApoE3 or ApoE2 genes.

Only five drugs have been approved by the FDA to treat Alzheimer's disease, and none of them stops or reverses the course of the disease. They have been shown to slow the worsening of the disease, but only for about six to twelve months on average, and only in about half the people who take them. Hundreds of drugs are currently in development for Alzheimer's, but it takes many millions of dollars and an average of thirteen years to bring a single drug from the concept stage to the market. Over the past few years, several promising vaccines and medications aimed at reducing the plaque in the brain have failed to show significant improvement in symptoms in people taking the drug. One such drug, Semagacestat from Eli Lilly, was even shown to cause accelerated worsening of the disease in people given the drug versus the placebo, as well as higher mortality and serious adverse effects in one in four people (Doody, 2013).

Even though the exact cause or causes of Alzheimer's disease are unknown, many details of its pathology have been worked out. The brain, which allows us to breathe and move and think, and defines who we are as individuals, is an incredibly complex machine, made up of a vast network of cells that interconnect with one another as well as to the other types of cells in the body. Hundreds of chemical reactions take place within each cell and cell membrane, and in the spaces between the cells where they connect and communicate with one another. These reactions are in delicate balance, and an excess or deficiency of one substance can upset this balance in such a way that the entire organ is affected. Insulin is one of those substances for which either an excess or a deficiency can have profoundly negative effects on the organ or organs involved. (This important idea is discussed in greater detail in Part Three.) When the balance of chemicals in the brain is upset, the unusual and the unexpected may occur as the caregivers of people with Alzheimer's can firmly attest to.

For more information on the possible causes of and contributors to Alzheimer's disease as well as the stages of Alzheimer's disease, see Appendices 2 and 3.

Mammy Staves Off Alzheimer's Disease

Catherine Frayne is Irish and a devoted daughter to her mother whom she calls Mammy. Her grandmother died with a constellation of symptoms that most likely represented Alzheimer's disease and, just as her Mammy reached her early eighties, she began to show similar symptoms, at first losing her keys and purse routinely, then jumping into the wrong car on more than one occasion and shopping twice for the same items. Her forgetfulness created anguish for her, and she began to overreact and have great difficulty coping. Her thinking and reasoning were not as sharp as before. Her geriatrician diagnosed her with a rapidly progressive form of Alzheimer's and his prognosis seemed to be on track as she deteriorated over the next several months and began to suffer from anxiety, became aggressive, and even threatened to harm her husband and others, all of which were highly uncharacteristic of Mammy.

Catherine would often take her mother out for the day to shop and go to a restaurant as she had always done. But now Catherine found that Mammy constantly repeated herself and asked the same questions over and over. While in the car she would pick up her purse, pull money out with great surprise, then put it back in and set the purse down, only to repeat the cycle moments later and again and again. After eating a full meal at a restaurant, upon leaving, she would tell Catherine she was hungry and ask when they were going to eat. She would also openly insult people while they were out. She stopped doing crossword puzzles, keeping lists, sewing, cooking, and doing laundry. She was obsessed with the idea that someone was robbing money from her, and Catherine soon discovered that Mammy was no longer keeping track of her finances. She continued to worsen and by early 2012 had lost interest in shopping and eating out. Her eyes appeared glazed, and she had lost the expression and animation in her face.

In February 2012, a friend sent Catherine a link to a YouTube video about coconut oil for Alzheimer's disease. The family began to give Mammy coconut oil, beginning with one teaspoon and increasing gradually. After two weeks they noticed that she was in a better mood and seemed to have a renewed interest in life. After a six-month hiatus, Catherine decided to take Mammy shopping again; her mother got herself up and ready for the trip and even called on the phone by herself to see if Catherine was on the way— something she had not been able to do for many months. After just a few weeks she became interested in watching the news, reading magazines, and gardening, and she began to cook, sew, and do laundry once again. She was brighter and more cheerful, initiating conversation more frequently. Four months after starting the coconut oil, on a visit with her doctor, her Mini-Mental Status Exam score was much improved to 25 out of 30 points and her clock drawing was now perfect. They told the doctor about the coconut oil and he said, "Whatever you are giving her, keep doing it because it's working. She is no longer a woman in decline."

Catherine has kept in touch and, more than two years later, she reports that her mother, now eighty-three, has continued to improve and is stable and doing very well. She has a great sense of humor, is still cooking and gardening of her own accord, and is back to writing lists to keep track of things. She is even back to doing crossword puzzles and sewing. Catherine Frayne has documented all of this in her beautifully and lovingly written book *Thoughts of Yesterday* (2013) (see www.CatherineFrayneAuthor.com).

Gloria's Husband Outlives Hospice Care

In 2010, I visited a nursing home north of Tampa in Florida to talk to caregivers and the staff about coconut oil and ketones for Alzheimer's and other dementias. Three years later I was invited to return and upon my arrival was greeted by a smiling Gloria, the wife of a nursing home patient who had been present for the previous talk. She and her husband are now in their early nineties and, in 2010, he was in the nursing home under hospice care. He has Alzheimer's disease, was cared for in bed, and was barely speaking. He was eating so poorly that he had lost more than 70 pounds and was down to 110 pounds. After my talk in 2010, Gloria began giving her husband coconut oil consistently with the help of the staff, and he gradually began to get out of bed, to have conversations, and to recognize her. His appetite improved so much that he regained fifty-five pounds and was dismissed from hospice care. He still resides at the nursing home, and Gloria spends the day with him. She showed me two pictures: one with her husband lying expressionless in bed from 2010; and the other more recent, showing him nicely dressed and sitting next to her, and both with lovely smiles on their faces.

Symptoms Are Arrested

E-mail sent by the husband of a woman with Alzheimer's disease on October 23, 2013: "J[oanne] has been on VCO [virgin coconut oil] now for 28 weeks and is much improved—we are doing seven tablespoons a day but not doing any of the other MCTs you mentioned. We are also planning to bring her home this Friday and will have a live-in 24/7 care. I'm excited and I think it will be helpful to Joanne also—her day-care nurse asked her if she was happy to be going home and she said, 'Now I have to deal with him. . . .' Thanks to you and VCO report we seem to have arrested things at least for the time being."

Three days later, on October 26, 2013, he writes: "Today is a milestone—after eight and a half months in a rehab facility and six and a half months on VCO, Joanne is revitalized—energized—alert—strong—healthy—engaged—can read—laughs a lot (what's new)—smiles—tries to talk but cannot always complete sentences—and [is] generally 100 percent better than she was on February 17, 2013 when she was very sick and weak. Yesterday, we left the nursing home and brought her home—we have a 24/7 day-care live-in who cooks and loves her—she worked at the facility where she [Joanne] was and knows her better than anyone at this point I think, so [she] decided she would like to continue to take care of Joanne at home—eight months ago I would not have thought this possible but it has happened and we have Dr. Mary to thank for that."

"K" Finds Her Words

E-mail received from the husband of a woman with early-onset Alzheimer's disease on January 23, 2014: "My wife, now sixty-three, is diagnosed with early-onset Alzheimer's disease since age sixty-two, although symptoms showed before that. After about one year on standard medications, we added coconut oil beginning in December 2013. It has made a difference, although "K" does not seem to realize it. Her speech is much better, way less searching for words. That started immediately and has continued to improve. Now she is more engaged socially, possibly because it is easier to talk. I am seeing some other improvements, less depression and frustration. Possibly some improvement in recall of older events. . . . This disease runs in her family, affecting her mother and also an older sister, although each one seems to show the effects at a younger age."

Mother Answers Phone Again

E-mail sent on February 21, 2014, from a Frenchwoman whose mother has Alzheimer's disease: "My mother has AD [Alzheimer's disease] at a serious level now, and I will try coconut oil with her, and me too." In a February 28, 2014 update, she writes: "After one week treatment, I'm so excited! I just finish a call with my mother! She first answer[ed] the phone, it was merely impossible one week ago, and she talked fluently to me! Finding words was merely impossible last week. The result is wonderful!" And in another update on March 12, 2014, she shares: "My mother laughed, she was happy, and did jokes. I was sooooooo happy to see her like that! Just with one small spoon at noon and evening, during fifteen days. She was speaking (much more) fluently, finding more words, and better memory and comprehension. Of course all is not perfect, lots of things are still difficult but really she is in great form compared to last month!"

8

Non-Alzheimer's Dementias

Dementia is a catchall term used to describe several different conditions that affect the brain. According to the online Free Dictionary, dementia is defined as "a loss of mental abilities severe enough to interfere with normal activities of daily living, lasting at least six months, not present from birth, and not associated with a loss or alteration of consciousness," and consists of a group of symptoms caused by the death of brain cells "leading to impairments in memory, reasoning, planning, and behavior" (www.thefreedictionary.com). Alzheimer's disease is the most common form of dementia, representing at least half of cases in the United States, but there are a number of other types of dementia, several of which we will discuss in this chapter. More detailed information about each of these disorders can be found on the website of the National Institutes of Health (NIH) division called the National Institute of Neurologic Disorders and Stroke (www.ninds.nih.gov).

The exact type or types of dementia cannot be determined with certainty without an autopsy at this time, so when a specific diagnosis is given when a person is alive it is a "best guess" based on imaging studies such as magnetic resonance imaging (MRI) scans and cognitive testing. Something all the dementias discussed here have in common, including vascular dementia, is the problem of decreased glucose uptake in the brain. Some of these diseases have been studied more than others with regard to whether this decrease in glucose uptake is the result of insulin resistance or some other factor. In any case, there may be little or nothing to lose by trying medium-chain triglycerides as coconut oil or MCT oil, since ketones produced by consuming them could potentially bypass the problem of getting glucose into the brain and into the affected brain cells.

LEWY BODY DEMENTIA: AN OFTEN MISDIAGNOSED DEMENTIA

According to the NIH pamphlet on *Lewy Body Dementia: Information for Patients, Families, and Professionals,* this form of dementia has jumped ahead of vascular dementia as the second most common after Alzheimer's, affecting more than 1.3 million Americans and representing about 20 percent of dementias worldwide. The NIH reports that many people with Lewy body dementia are misdiagnosed as having Alzheimer's disease, but that some people with this condition also have Alzheimer's or Parkinson's. As opposed to the plaques and tangles found in people with Alzheimer's disease, those with Lewy body dementia have abnormal deposits of a protein called alpha-synuclein in the brain that affect thinking, movement, behavior, and mood. Lewy body dementia has gained wider recognition since the sudden suicide death in 2014 of famous actor Robin Williams who was diagnosed with Parkinson's disease but found at time of autopsy to actually suffer from Lewy body dementia.

People with Lewy bodies tend to have cognitive decline similar to those with Alzheimer's disease. But they also develop other symptoms including severe rapid eye movement (REM) sleep disturbances, such as night terrors (acting out dreams); visual hallucinations in 80 percent (often seeing little people and animals that aren't there); fluctuations in attention, alertness, and cognitive abilities; and Parkinson-type movement problems, such as stiffness and slow movement. They are often very sensitive to medications, such as antipsychotics, resulting in serious adverse reactions, and many develop symptoms of depression, apathy, anxiety, agitation, paranoia, and/or delusions (false beliefs). Certain medications used to try to treat these symptoms, such antipsychotics, antidepressants, and benzodiazepines, can make some people with this disease worse. There is no known cure for the disease itself.

Condition Stabilizes

Helga Rohra is a German author and now a speaker on the subject of dementia, who was diagnosed with Lewy body dementia in 2007. Steve, our daughter Joanna, and I got to know Helga at the Alzheimer's Disease International Conference in Greece in 2010 for which I was an invited speaker on coconut oil and ketones as an alternative fuel for Alzheimer's. Helga took the idea of using coconut oil to heart and has reported to me that she continues to use coconut oil in her diet and her disease has been quite stable. In fact, she wrote the foreword to the German translation of my book, which was published in 2013!

Vacant Look Gone

E-mail sent by the wife of a man with Lewy body dementia on August 17, 2013: "I wanted to let you know that I have seen great improvement in my husband since I started giving him coconut oil. He is more engaged in conversation, doing chores, and the typical things he used to do around the house. He also got back his sense of humor and the vacant look in his eyes is all but gone. Having said all of the above, he still has the 'Capgras' delusion problem and still gets a little confused." Capgras syndrome is a failure to recognize a very significant person in one's life, such as the spouse-caregiver, while still recognizing others.

Positive Change

E-mail received from the son of a seventy-four-year-old man with Lewy body dementia and Parkinson's disease on June 27, 2014: "Since [my father began] taking the coconut oil, I have noticed a positive change in his mobility; his personality is starting to come back; and at times his thinking is clearer, which is progress in comparison to where he was just a few weeks ago. We are still working on the amount he can tolerate but we are happy with the results."

VASCULAR DEMENTIA: A CEREBROVASCULAR DEMENTIA

In vascular dementia, inflammation and narrowing of the arteries that carry blood to the brain results in damage to the areas served by them. Some people with vascular dementia have a series of small strokes (called multi-infarct dementia), and new symptoms may appear suddenly when these strokes occur. Risk factors for vascular dementia include a history of strokes or mini-strokes, heart attacks, atherosclerosis (hardening of the arteries), high blood pressure, diabetes, smoking, and atrial fibrillation (an abnormal heart rhythm that can cause a blood clot to form in the heart).

Vascular dementia as the sole cause of dementia accounts for about 10 percent of all dementias, however, many people (about 50 percent of the total with dementia) have evidence of both vascular dementia and one or more other types of dementia, most commonly Alzheimer's disease, in which case the condition is called a "mixed dementia." In 1906, Alois Alzheimer, a German psychiatrist and neuropathologist, first reported the disease which eventually was given his name in a fifty-one-year-old woman, Auguste Deter, noting the plaques and tangles in her brain after she died that are now considered to be the hallmarks of the disease. However, he also found signs of hardening of the arteries, indicative of the overlap often seen between vascular dementia and Alzheimer's disease.

Alzheimer's medications often have a similar response in people with vascular dementia. Drugs to prevent blood clotting are often prescribed as are strategies to reduce the risk by controlling diabetes and high blood pressure, and encouraging smoking cessation.

The First Twenty-Four Hours

Ethelle Lord is a pioneer in Alzheimer's coaching and is the founder of Remembering 4 You (www.Remembering4You.com) and the International Caregivers Association, a distance dementia-training association. She is the author of *How in the World . . . And Now What Do I Do? A Primer for Alzheimer's: 12 Major Points for Coping Better* (2013) and the forthcoming book *Alzheimer's Coaching: Taking a Systems Approach to Creating an Alzheimer's Friendly Healthcare Workforce* (2015). She first contacted me by e-mail not long after her husband responded positively to coconut oil in 2012 and, when I asked for follow-up she kindly provided me with this detailed account.

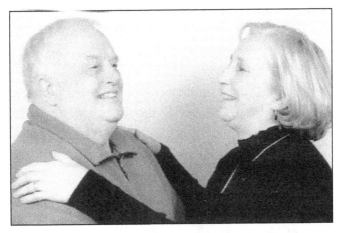

FIGURE 8.1. Ethelle Lord and Major Larry S. Potter

On April 5, 2014, she writes: "My husband, Major Larry S. Potter, retired U.S. Air Force, is a twenty-one-year veteran of the military, a retired business professor, and a wonderful man. In the fall of 1999, he underwent emergency triple bypass surgery in Boston and had a normal recovery, except for one major problem: every time he went up a set of stairs, he would fall; and every time he started walking down a hall, he could not stop himself from running until he hit a wall. With each fall he hurt his knees, and as a result he became fearful of walking. A researcher from Harvard Medical School informed me that my husband's brain must have been traumatized as a result of the heart surgery and that it had nothing to do with dementia.

"His recovery proceeded normally and he returned to teach at the University of Maine in Presque Isle within a few months. I am not a medical doctor, but even though I could see that physically he had recovered from the heart surgery, I could also see that he was becoming more and more tired and more and more forgetful. I won't go into details, but he would do things as forget to do his errands on the way home from teaching classes.

"On the afternoon of January 30, 2003 (a date that will live in infamy in our family), his doctor finally informed both of us that he suspected Larry had Alzheimer's disease. So many other millions of families have such a date, too. He was subsequently diagnosed with vascular dementia by a cardiologist at a Veterans Affairs medical center.

"Life unfolded as it should with his vascular dementia. More and more it became difficult for him to speak, both in finding the right words and in completing his sentences. I remember his saying something one day that did not make any sense or reason. He simply turned to me and said, 'Forget what I just said. It makes no sense.' This kind of awareness in him in spite of the dementia was remarkable.

"We are told that eventually everything will go: memories, voice, and recognizing even close family members. So as I recommend to everyone who receives such a diagnosis, early on I recorded both his voice for myself and my voice for him, so that should he end up in long-term care someday, hearing my voice might be of comfort to him.

"About 80 percent of individuals living with Alzheimer's disease or dementia end up in long-term care. Mostly this is because after years of homecare, pack leaders (family caregivers) are completely worn out physically, emotionally, and financially. After Larry was placed in long-term care, his speech continued to deteriorate and also diminish considerably. It came to the point at which I no longer heard him speak. I knew that inside he was still the same man with lots of thoughts, feelings, and ideas, but what I missed the most was hearing his voice. And I feared that his care was compromised because he was unable to ask for what he wanted, to say how he felt, and to refuse to do what he did not care to do. It was a very stressful time for us, especially for me as his primary caregiver and pack leader. He went from being able only to scream when he was turned in bed to being silent.

"In the late fall of 2012, I was doing research for my small business, Remembering 4 You, and came across a short series of videos on YouTube of Dr. Mary Newport who was being interviewed with her husband, Steve (www.youtube.com/watch?v=iScs0uzQZFk). These videos changed our lives forever. I immediately purchased coconut oil (the extra-virgin type) and took it to my husband. Another famous date for me is December 23, 2012: the day I gave my husband his first two tablespoons of coconut oil. The next day, less than 24 hours after the first two tablespoons, and after a total of only six tablespoons, he called me by my first name, Ethelle, the most warming word out of his mouth after over a year of silence.

"Soon after that day he asked me, 'Are you happy?' as I entered his room. Wow! I was about on my knees by then, and realized the power of coconut oil in the best possible way. Larry was able to speak—to speak his mind, and he was back!

"The first day I introduced coconut oil into Larry's diet, the doctor and nursing staff thought I was crazy. They even had a meeting about adding coconut oil to his regimen and decided that the doctor had to prescribe it. His doctor, an old-fashioned Maine country doctor, concluded that coconut oil was a food, not a prescription drug, and that it could not hurt considering the advanced condition of Larry's vascular dementia.

"Since that first 24 hours at Christmastime in 2012, my husband has not stopped asking for what he wants, saying how he feels, and refusing to do what he does not care to do. This is enormous considering he is dependent on others for his total care. It was especially comforting to me to be able to leave him after visits knowing he would be able to 'defend' himself with more than moans and groans.

"Larry recently suffered with a *Clostridium difficile* infection. *C. difficile* releases toxins that cause bloating, diarrhea, and serious and severe abdominal pain, and compromises the entire digestive system. Many do not survive a *C. difficile* infection no matter their age. It mimics the flu and can last for several weeks to months. In Larry's case, I believe that having been on coconut oil for over a year helped his body successfully fight this infection due to coconut oil's natural antimicrobial, antibacterial, antifungal, and antioxidant properties (wellnessmama.com/2072/benefits-of-coconut-oil).

"Because of the *C. difficile* infection, we had to replace the coconut oil with medium-chain triglyceride (MCT) oil for a short time. Coconut oil therapy requires that enzymes from the intestines be absorbed into the body. Because Larry's digestive system was completely compromised by the *C. difficile,* and after consulting with Dr. Newport, it made sense for him to switch to MCT oil to preserve his ketone level as much as possible during his illness. I also added essential oregano oil to the reflexology therapy [a type of therapeutic massage] I gave him to support him further in fighting this deadly infection. After two months of confinement to his room with C. *difficile,* he came out of this health crisis in a remarkable way.

"I now keep coconut oil close at hand because it is the single most important of all his supplements. I also use it for cooking in recipes I prepare for us. (When I travel I take along coconut oil to stay regular, and I use it on my skin with a few drops of essential oil.) To this day, and with the introduction of other supplements to his diet, I can say that he continues to make progress and his symptoms are reversing thanks to those first 24 hours."

Wicked Sense of Humor Returns

E-mail sent from the caregiver for a woman with vascular dementia on December 9, 2011: "Now, after a year of taking coconut oil, she is much brighter in herself, more interested in her surroundings and can speak better. She is now feeding herself again, albeit, with a spoon, but that's great. She understands nearly everything that we say. I feel that she is trapped inside her body, understanding what is going on but is unable to find the words to speak to us properly, and is not always able to control her body as she would like. This must be so frustrating. . . . Life for me is much better now, at least I can have partial conversations with her. Her wicked sense of humour [humor] has come back and she enjoys a good joke. If I tease her or anyone else, I get severely reprimanded by her. If she did not understand this, I certainly would not do it."

Man Loses Sweet Tooth, Finds Conversation

E-mail sent by the son of a seventy-nine-year-old man with vascular dementia and Alzheimer's disease on February 21, 2012: "Some of the changes we have noticed in my dad are:

1. Participating in conversations.

2. Initiating conversations.

3. Forming complete sentences.

4. Return of his personality.

5. No longer fixating on sweets and sugar.

6. Interested in getting back on his computer. Note: this will require a bit of training."

No Longer Confuses Mouthwash with Shampoo

E-mail received from the wife of an eighty-five-year-old man with strokes and vascular dementia on May 18, 2012: "He had two strokes in 2010 which has [have] led to vascular dementia and has only partial movement on the right side and double vision. His mental function has been on a steady decline. I started him on coconut oil April 19, 2012. Two hours after giving him the coconut oil he stood up by himself with no assistance. This was the first time he was able to do this since after his fall in January 2012. He has not forgotten my name once since the coconut oil—he has not called me "Mom" and thought I was his mother. His short-term memory is improved—he can, at times, now remember things from three days previously. He can on occasion speak in full sentences (not always but he has not spoke[n] in complete sentences since November 2010). His sense of humor is back, he has not confused his mouthwash with shampoo—for some reason he was constantly trying to put mouthwash on his hair. His word finding has improved. He has a more alert look in his eyes, he is able to do some things which take multi steps without cues he could not do before."

Four days later, on May 22, 2012, I received the following update:

"I believe the coconut is still working and I am seeing little bits of improving. There is not a doubt in my mind or his that the coconut oil is helping his cognitive [cognition]. His memory is so improved, today he reminded me of something from four days ago, which I had forgotten. Prior to the coconut oil this would not have happened. I missed the oil one day, and he went into almost a stupor. I thought perhaps he had a TIA [transient ischemic attack], but when I realized I had forgotten the oil, I gave him a dose. He took a nap and when he woke up, the color was back in his face and light back in his eyes."

FRONTOTEMPORAL DEMENTIA: A DEMENTIA THAT AFFECTS PERSONALITY AND LANGUAGE

Frontotemporal dementia (FTD) was called Pick's disease for many years after it was first described by physician Arnold Pick in 1892. FTD accounts for 10 to 15 percent of dementias overall. This disease involves atrophy (shrinkage) and dysfunction of brain cells in the frontal and/or temporal areas of the brain that are involved in speaking and understanding speech, planning and organization, judgment, emotions, and certain types of movement, but memory impairment is not usually part of the problem, at least early on.

There are several different forms of this disease depending on which symptoms are most prominent. For people in whom the language centers are most involved, the disease is referred to as primary progressive aphasia, in which the person may either have difficulty generating words, or as semantic dementia, in which the individual may substitute incorrect words and have difficulty conveying what he or she means to say. For others with the behavioral variant of FTD, the parts of the brain involved in behavior and personality are most affected and they often become uninhibited or impulsive, and exhibit inappropriate social behavior and a lack of empathy, while others may become listless and bored, and may suffer from depression as well.

Two other forms of FTD involve involuntary and automatic movement that may or may not affect language and behavior. One form is called corticobasal degeneration, which involves shakiness, lack of coordination, muscles spasms, and stiffness; the other is known as progressive supranuclear palsy, which causes abnormal eye movements, stiffness in the neck and upper body, and problems with walking and balance.

Eventually, people with this group of FTD diseases are unable to speak; they become bedbound and their life span is generally shortened as a result of the disease. As in several of the other dementias previously mentioned, accumulations of abnormal proteins appear to be involved and only symptomatic treatments are available, which usually include antidepressants and anticonvulsants, none of which are approved by the FDA to treat FTD.

Independence Regained

The wife of a seventy-eight-year-old man with FTD writes on December 2, 2008: "I read your article on the use of coconut oil; I also read that the Food and Drug Administration approved the drug Axona . . . and would like to try him on the drug. . . . He has improved significantly with the coconut oil." [I suggested she purchase MCT oil while waiting for Axona to be available, and I asked her for more information and to keep in touch about her husband's progress. Over the next months, she experimented with giving her husband the oils individually or in combination and eventually increased dosing from once to three times a day.]

Three weeks later, on December 23, 2008, she writes: "My husband's memory has improved and his ability to speak and recall words is better. He has been taking MCT oil now for about a month, three tablespoons in the morning. What hasn't improved is his ability to make good decisions."

Nearly six weeks later, on February 1, 2009, she followed up: "I decided to try just MCT oil, three tablespoons in the morning, but then I noticed that in the late afternoon he started to fade out on me. So I started giving him one tablespoon in the afternoon and he was better. I think he did much better on the coconut oil so I have switched him back to the coconut oil. I am still using some MCT oil."

Just short of four months, on May 19, 2009, she sent the following update: "Taking the oil three times a day in the proportion you suggested [four teaspoons of MCT oil, plus three teaspoons of coconut oil]. I started him on the oil [five months ago] because of bizarre behavior, such as giving away thousands of dollars, melting a Netflix video in the toaster oven (because he needed to dry it), and putting a dishtowel in the microwave and causing a fire. Since I started him on the oil he has not exhibited this bizarre behavior. He still has problems but not as severe. . . . Since I started him on the oil, and especially now that he is taking it three times a day, he has improved dramatically. . . . I am assuming the oil works just as well with frontotemporal dementia, since his behavior has improved."

Two months later, on July 12, 2009, I received the following: "He is not perfect, but he is very independent . . ."

Temperament Improves

E-mail sent by the wife of a man with FTD on February 10, 2012: "I started him on the MCT oil. Each day I see some improvement. His temperament has improved 99 percent (which is where he was before), he can draw a much better circle, his eating habits have improved 4-fold, his speech also has improved, and his communication with others has too. All are improvements even before the coconut oil. . . . I will see what the next month brings and how he is progressing, but a 20 percent improvement is better than nothing at all!"

Even Late-Stage Dementia Responds

E-mail received from the husband of a woman with late-stage FTD on March 19, 2013: "My wife, age seventy-one, has late-stage FTD and has been on coconut oil for about four weeks. It has helped her come back a little. No miracle, but she is again making eye contact with me and verbalizing again. She is more responsive. I am definitely continuing the treatment."

9

Parkinson's Disease

Parkinson's disease was first described in 1817 by the English surgeon James Parkinson. At least 500,000 people in the United States suffer from the disease, although this may be a gross underestimate. Symptoms begin to appear after 60 to 80 percent of the cells that produce the important hormone–neurotransmitter dopamine have died in an area of the brain called the substantia nigra. Dopamine has many effects throughout the body and brain, but when this area of the brain is involved, movement is most affected. The disease slowly but progressively worsens, usually over a period of many years, and most people with Parkinson's do not die as a direct result of the disease, although it results in very significant disability. The average age at onset is sixty, but 5 to 10 percent have the early-onset form of the disease—notably, the actor Michael J. Fox, who has established a foundation to learn more about the disease and to find treatments.

Like Lewy body dementia, people with Parkinson's disease have abnormal deposits of the protein alpha-synuclein in brain cells called Lewy bodies. They also have dysfunction of the mitochondria (organelles inside all cells that produce the final energy molecule ATP), oxidative stress, and inflammation in the brain. Recent evidence points to a significant role for insulin resistance in Parkinson's disease and a link with type 2 diabetes. Upward of 50 to 80 percent of people with Parkinson's also show glucose intolerance when tested and, like people with Alzheimer's, there is decreased glucose uptake in the affected parts of the brain. The most commonly used drug to treat Parkinson's disease, levodopa (L-dopa), tends to abnormally raise blood sugar and increase insulin resistance; so, the drug may treat the symptoms but potentially can make matters worse for the long haul (Aviles-Olmos, 2013).

PARKINSON'S DISEASE: A NEURODEGENERATIVE DISEASE

Parkinson's disease is a movement disorder in which the person develops problems with tremors, muscle stiffness, and cramps, hesitation when initiating walking, and sudden freezing while walking. People with Parkinson's often have reduced facial expression and animation (called "masked face"), may speak softly, have stooped posture, slow movement, problems with balance and coordination with a tendency to fall and a shuffling of the feet when walking. Many suffer from depression and sleep problems, such as restless leg syndrome and night terrors. Eventually, they develop problems with swallowing and chewing, which may seriously affect nutrition and make them prone to aspirating food. When someone with Parkinson's disease develops dementia, the problems with movement typically appear at least one year before the cognitive problems, and the person often goes on to develop problems with mood, behavior, and cognition.

While for most people the exact cause of Parkinson's is unknown, there are a few known causes of the disease. There was a marked increase in Parkinson's following a worldwide epidemic of a virus that caused encephalitis (inflammation of the brain) in 5 million people following World War I; a chemical called MPTP (1-methyl-4-phenyl-1,2,3,6-tetrahydropyridine) developed to treat heroin addiction in the 1980s had the unexpected side effect of severe permanent Parkinson's disease as a result of killing off brain cells that produce dopamine; and certain drugs to treat psychosis (and often used against FDA guidelines in Alzheimer's patients), such as haloperidol (Haldol) and chlorpromazine (Thorazine), may cause Parkinson's symptoms that are usually, but not always, reversible when stopped.

There is no drug available that will cure Parkinson's disease. Certain drugs that increase or mimic dopamine or keep it from breaking down and other treatments, such as a surgically implanted deep brain stimulator (a device similar to a pacemaker that sends electrical pulses to the relevant area of the brain), may improve symptoms. Exercise and a healthy whole-food diet that is naturally high in antioxidants could help as well. Recent research suggests that treatments for type 2 diabetes may also be beneficial in Parkinson's disease (Aviles-Olmos, 2013).

Reports from People with Parkinson's Disease

I have received numerous reports from people with Parkinson's disease who believe they have improved while taking coconut oil or MCT oil or a combination (such as in Fuel for Thought).

In 2005, Dr. VanItallie and his colleagues published a report of five people with Parkinson's disease who were able to adhere strictly to a classic ketogenic diet (90 percent of calories as fat, 8 percent as protein, 2 percent as carbohydrate) for a twenty-eight-day period and go into ketosis, as verified by increased ketone levels as well as lower glucose and insulin levels (VanItallie, 2005). At the end of the twenty-eight days, the people experienced a 43.4 percent improvement, ranging from 21 to 81 percent based on the Unified Parkinson's Disease Rating Scale (UPDRS), a test that rates the symptoms of Parkinson's disease. The researchers found improvements in resting tremor, freezing, balance, gait, mood, and energy level.

More than thirty people have reported to me that the relatively mild increase in ketone levels from consuming coconut or MCT oil or both has resulted in similar improvements. A few have reported improvement followed by stabilization for two years or longer. One man with Parkinson's disease, who felt that he had improvement from coconut oil but too much fluctuation between doses, found success with the ketogenic diet, another option to consider. The ketogenic diet is discussed in more detail in Chapter 13.

Dr. VanItallie, who developed Fuel for Thought, an MCT oil-enriched coconut oil, to treat people with Parkinson's and Alzheimer's, as well as other neurodegenerative diseases, has received testimonials from many others of improvement.

Every Day I Feel Better

E-mail received from a lady with Parkinson's disease on December 9, 2013: "I'm a sixty-five-year-old female, diagnosed with Parkinson's disease in January 2001. I had seen some YouTube videos about coconut oil and Alzheimer's and wondered about benefits to PD [Parkinson's disease] patients. I began to read up on other health benefits of coconut oil and wanted to add it to my diet, but couldn't find an appealing way to get tablespoons of coconut oil down without gagging. I started introducing small amounts into my food with absolutely no effect. I finally learned by liquefying the coconut oil first and dribbling it into a blender with a breakfast shake, I could add at least two or three tablespoons without being able to detect it. The first day I put two tablespoons in my breakfast shake was a really great day. It was unusual that I didn't need a nap, and I remember just feeling better but writing it off as a coincidence. I wish I would have noted the date, but I didn't suspect the significance.

"It's been about three weeks and every day I feel better. The crippling PD fatigue is very substantially changed for the better. Previously, the fatigue worsened my posture, voice, and energy. Friends and family have already begun to comment on what they describe as startling changes in my appearance, volume of my voice, and overall look of improved health. I was hoping that coconut oil might slow the progression of PD, but I wasn't expecting short-term noticeable improvement. To realize an immediate benefit that feels very substantial is exhilarating. I don't know whether coconut oil enhances the absorption [of] other supplements like the [coenzyme] Q10 or whether my particular physical deficiencies are receptive to the unique properties within coconut oil, but I know the difference in the way I feel. For the last few years when asked how I feel, I always gave the same enthusiastic response, "I'm hanging in there!" Now, my response is, "I'm feeling *great!*" I urge anybody curious about whether coconut oil might help with PD symptoms to give it a try. After being diagnosed so long ago, I could have never dreamed such a simple and yummy remedy could impact my life so much."

On April 3, 2014, about five months after she started using coconut oil, I received this update: "I am doing great, thank you. I am absolutely still on coconut oil. I'm afraid not to take it for a single day. I take 2 to 3 tablespoons in a morning shake every day. I don't take CO in the afternoon because it makes me feel like doing other things instead of sleeping. Though I still have PD, my life is greatly improved. I can do so many small things now that used to cause me great difficulty. Buttoning my pants, cutting my meat, standing on one leg to put on my pants, speaking louder, walking quickly. . . . I don't want to forget how much difference coconut oil makes or to take its benefits for granted. My new doctor actually seemed irritated that I attributed the undeniable improvement to coconut oil. He tested and rated my PD on my initial visit with him, which coincidentally was just a few weeks before I started coconut oil. I asked if he would repeat the tests for comparisons, but he declined. I'm looking for a new neurologist. FYI: In addition, I begged my niece to put my older sister, who has Alzheimer's, on coconut oil. She also had dramatic improvement. Within the first four days she was interacting with her family again, even going to lunch and a movie. After twelve years of not being able to have any meaningful phone conversations with her, we now converse regularly and she sounds the way she did fifteen years ago. What's more, my younger sister has diabetes, heart disease, [and] fibromyalgia. Since she has been on 4 tablespoons of coconut oil per day, she has cut her insulin in half, she has increased energy, and she has lost over 50 lbs."

Something Real Has Happened To Me

E-mail received from Wes Wilson, a man in his seventies with Parkinson's disease on May 31, 2013: "I am seventy-four years old and I have Parkinson's, diagnosed $3^1/_2$ years ago and under conventional treatment by Mayo Clinic. A year ago, while taking Mirapex ER (3 mg) and Azilect (1 mg), my symptoms had progressed to severe slowness, unsteadiness, chronic stiffness and joint pain, frequent freezing episodes and I dragged my left leg. I had lost all facial expression and my left leg was retaining a significant amount of fluid (swelling to about 150 percent). The addition of carbidopa/levodopa (25/100 [mg], 3 per day) eased the joint pain and the freezing episodes and restored some of the lost balance, but I still had annoying unsteadiness, slow movement, and could not rise from a low chair unassisted. I still dragged my left leg.

"This past April, I began taking coconut oil, worked up to 4 tablespoons daily (2 with breakfast, 1 at lunch, 1 at dinner). I saw significant improvements in a couple of days. My wife and friends are astonished at my apparent recovery. It is strikingly noticeable. The reason for this dosage pattern is that I can feel a return of old symptoms 6–8 hours after the last dose.

"Current status:

- I move so quickly about the house (kitchen) that my wife and I collide.

- My speed on the elliptical trainer changed from 2.0 mph to 3.5 mph in a few days (I had to be careful with this, my knees were not used to this level of performance).

- I can do the DUI tests [driving sobriety tests] (close eyes, stand on one foot, etc.).

- I can rise from any chair unassisted.

- I can do football agility drills (shift right, shift left, step forward, step back in response to random commands).

- Past and present photos show a pronounced change in facial expression.

- I can smell again.

- My osteopath has noticed a pronounced improvement in joint flexibility.

- The swelling in my left leg has disappeared.

- I walk normally, but still have a tendency to stoop.

- My primary care physician has declared my improvement miraculous, he calls me his 'clinical trial of one.'

"I have no delusions that this is a cure. I still have Parkinson's symptoms, but my quality of life has vastly improved. We are about at the end of 2 months [after starting the coconut oil], and the benefits are maintaining. Something real has happened to me, and I applaud your dedication to publicizing the benefits of coconut oil."

Four and one-half months later, on September 16, 2013, I received an update from Wes. He reported that he has been taking eight tablespoons of coconut oil daily (two with breakfast, two at lunch, two at dinner, two at bedtime). He also sent me pictures of himself walking along a series of railroad ties (Figure 9.1) along with this poem:

RAILROAD TIES

PD* can debilitate	8T CO** is what it takes
If you wonder,	Add 1,000 calories,
I'm Feeling Great	Still lose weight?
Walk Railroad ties	Learn to spurn
with a steady gait	Carbohydrates.

* PD = Parkinson's disease   ** CO = Coconut oil

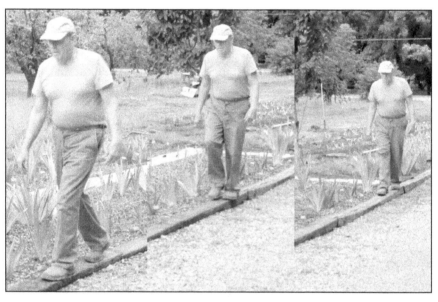

FIGURE 9.1. Wes Wilson's balance improved so much after taking coconut oil for four months that he was able to walk along railroad ties.

On his website Wes states: "I fear that the poetic line 'Learn to spurn Carbohydrates' may have been taken too literally. I include carbohydrates in my diet, and do not advocate a ketogenic diet except for those who are operating with medical advice and medical supervision. In my diet I receive carbohydrates from skim milk, green leafy vegetables, beans, and a limited amount of whole grain. I spurn foods with a high glycemic index: sugar, white starches, almost anything with corn or corn products, ripe banana, and concentrated fruit juice."

On January 15, 2015, I heard again from Wes and here are excerpts from the letter: "I am older. I see signs of aging and I notice that Parkey is making some gains. Not exactly measurable, since my UPDRS score actually reduced in each of the last two years. For physical evidence, several people who have administered physical therapy to me commented that they can feel the increasing flexibility of my muscles shortly after I take a dose of coconut oil. One who is watching me closely has noted a gradual increase in stiffening of the muscles between doses. As I get further from the time of the last dose, I notice an increase in stiffening and pain [in] some large muscle groups, which goes away in a few minutes after taking my next coconut oil. The model in my mind is that I am increasing the level of an essential nutrient (ketones) and the tapering is similar to the reaction to reduced blood sugar that we all experience if we go too long between meals. We eat carbohydrates to increase our blood sugar, which works for a while and then must be refurbished. I eat CO to increase ketones, which I need. My intellectual model is that it is all nutritional for me. I am happy to say that I still get a substantial benefit from CO. Two years ago I was nearly crippled from PD. For the past two years I have been quite functional and it continues. My doctor and I think it is the nutritional benefit. Others may choose to call it placebo, witchcraft, or whatever. That is their right. For me it works and continues to work."

Wes developed a format to document changes for people with Parkinson's disease while taking coconut oil and has also collected case reports with the goal of convincing Parkinson's associations to study this dietary intervention. For more information, see http://tending-the-iris.us/coconut-oil-benefits-for-parkinsons-disease.

It's Almost a Miracle

E-mail received from a child whose father has Parkinson's disease and dementia on November 26, 2012: "I have my ninety-year-old father with late-stage dementia on coconut oil. It's almost a miracle. . . . The day after he started, he began walking without his walker with his hands in his pockets, like the old days! He was alert, awake, and more animated. He was able to speak a few more words than in the past. We thought it was a placebo effect [. . .]. Then he ran out of the oil for one week [. . .] he was *so* bad, his legs locked (he does have Parkinson's and is on Mirapex, he couldn't walk at all!! He also didn't laugh, didn't talk, couldn't feed himself, and he was staring into space again. Immediately restarted the oil, and within 24 hours (honestly), he was laughing, responding to others, saying 3–4 word sentences, acting more like himself, and walking again! I can hardly believe it, and if I hadn't seen it with my own eyes, I wouldn't believe it!"

No Medication, Only Fuel for Thought

E-mail received from a man with Parkinson's disease on September 21, 2013: "About 3 years ago I was diagnosed with PD. Mostly it was a tremor in my right arm. I had some problems swallowing and noticed an increase in saliva. I am taking no medication at this time and see a neurologist twice a year. On April 12, 2013, I started taking Fuel for Thought. I take one vial in the morning and one in the afternoon. I have kept up this on a regular basis. I noticed that my problem with swallowing disappeared and also my problem with saliva. My tremor has decreased and mostly occurs when I am under stress. My wife has commented on this also. My balance is OK although I had a hip replaced last year."

The Power of a Low-Carb Diet and Coconut Oil

E-mail sent by a sixty-five-year-old man with Parkinson's and memory impairment on December 8, 2013: "Up until four years ago I had gradually developed tremors in my hands, sometime my foot would drag on the toe area as I walked, and my balance was suffering; I thought this was just normal age progression. I also increasingly needed longer and longer naps, and after sleeping a full night would go back to bed at around 11:00 a.m. for a couple of hours. I noticed my memory declining, along with more difficulty in pulling up words from my brain. (Incidentally, I worked as an accountant, like your husband, before I retired.) . . . Last spring I decided to lose weight, as at 5'11" I was obese at 245 lbs. I had read the book *Wheat Belly* written by a cardiologist and decided to eliminate all grains from my diet and just eat meat (mostly steaks and pork chops), green vegetables, and Atkins' shakes and keep my calories under 1,500 a day. As my weight loss progressed, I stumbled upon the ketogenic diet, and as a result, increased the fat content of my diet. In order to increase fat I added coconut oil, butter, and bacon plus more cheese. My wife read about intermittent fasting, and we both began also to limit our caloric intake to 500 calories two successive days a week, and I simply ate four tablespoons of coconut oil on those days. The result on my shaky hands was to almost totally eliminate what shaking that remained. . . . I also walk faster, and my balance is much improved. While it is subjective, I experience my thinking as being much clearer."

Amyotrophic Lateral Sclerosis

A myotrophic lateral sclerosis, or ALS, is another nightmare of a neurodegenerative disease that involves the loss of motor neurons (nerve cells that control movement) in the spine, cerebral cortex, and brain stem, leading to progressive weakness. Fifty percent of people suffering with this disease die within three years after diagnosis, and 90 percent by five years, usually from respiratory failure. The average age of onset is fifty-five, but ALS can develop in much younger people. More than 22,000 people in the United States are living with ALS.

ALS: A PROGRESSIVE PARALYZING DISEASE

ALS is more commonly known as Lou Gehrig's disease, for the famous baseball player who succumbed to the disease in 1941. Early on, the person with ALS will have weakness in one or more parts of the body, such as the hands or legs. Gradually, the muscles atrophy or shrink, causing cramping, spasms, stiffness, and sometimes fasciculations (muscle twitches). There is no loss of touch or other sensations with ALS, and the afflicted person usually retains full awareness and other cognitive functions throughout the course of the disease. Eventually, as the disease progresses, the muscle weakness becomes so severe that the person loses complete independence and requires total care. When someone with ALS reaches the stage where he or she can no longer talk, swallow, or breathe effectively, difficult decisions have to be made regarding whether to provide nutrition by using a feeding tube inserted through the mouth or the stomach (a gastrostomy), and to assist breathing with a ventilator.

Like many other neurodegenerative diseases, a crucial part of the problem in ALS is abnormal glucose uptake into brain and nerve cells (Van Laere, 2014). Thus ketones could provide alternative fuel to these cells and potentially lessen the effects of the disease.

Much like Alzheimer's disease, the cause or causes of ALS are not certain and there is no medication on the market at present that will prevent, stop, or reverse the disease process.

Clarence Gets the Upper Hand in His Battle with ALS

Clarence Machlan was fifty-eight years old when he began to see signs in himself of familial ALS and was officially diagnosed a year later in 2008. He inherited this disease from his mother, who lived with the condition for eight years. For the first year Clarence did nothing special to try to treat his disease because he was told by his doctors, and then believed himself, that there was nothing he could do.

A year later, in the fall of 2009, Clarence read some things that lead him to wonder what did he have to lose by thinking outside the box. He first began taking a magnesium chloride and water mixture to counteract the many problems associated with magnesium deficiency, and about six weeks later began taking coconut oil. He started with four tablespoons a day and then worked up gradually over several months to three tablespoons, three times a day, mixed into food for a total of nine tablespoons per day. Just over a year later he also began to massage coconut oil into his "bad leg," twice a day, and saw an increase of three-eighth's inches in his thigh measurement, as well as an increase in strength over the next six weeks.

He first wrote to me about fourteen months after starting coconut oil to thank me and to tell me what had happened, and has updated me periodically thereafter.

As mentioned, people with ALS are expected to steadily deteriorate. Clarence wrote that, several months after beginning this regimen, he realized that rather than deteriorating further he actually had experienced some slight improvement, and that this progress continued. The changes were slow but in the right direction. Here are the changes he reported that occurred between September 15, 2009 and April 3, 2012:

- While he continued to require canes or crutches to walk due to weakness in his right leg, this right leg no longer felt "asleep" and was somewhat more responsive when walking.

- The circumference of his right thigh had increase by $1^3/_8$ inches and his left thigh by $1^1/_2$ inches.

- He had increased strength in both legs and could no longer feel the bones through his shrunken thigh muscles; he could push his right leg down with some force, which he could not do at all before taking coconut oil.

- He had gained almost five pounds from 148 to 152.9.

- His score on an ALS functional rating test had improved by 5 percent.

- While he still had foot drop in his right foot due to ankle weakness, it was only slight now.

- He was now able to tip his right foot up and down and side to side, and could move his toes up and down better than before.

- He was now able to raise his right thigh to put on his pants while sitting and had much less difficulty putting on his right shoe.

- His right ankle no longer appeared bruised whereas before it was purple almost all the way around.

- He went from having extreme difficulty rolling over in bed to rolling over with a minimum of effort.

- He previously had trouble with thick and excess saliva at night, but this was no longer a problem.

- He had mild insomnia and would get up to use the restroom twice during the night but now sleeps better and almost never needs to get up.

- He had completely stopped having cramps and spasms in both legs.

- He no longer had weakness in either hand.

- Electromyograms (EMGs) done a year apart in 2011 and 2012 showed "no changes," which is unusual for someone with ALS; his doctors began to doubt their diagnosis but told him to keep doing what he was doing.

In an update in 2013 at four years after starting his regimen, Clarence reported that he continues to massage his leg with coconut oil once a day and is still taking nine tablespoons of coconut oil per day. He has no new symptoms and has continued to gain strength in his legs, fingers, hands, and arms. He has improved so much that his doctors decided to go forward with knee replacement surgery for a problem unrelated to his ALS, and he was doing well following the surgery. He still walks with the assistance of crutches but is able to drive when necessary. He told me that once a year he tries stopping the coconut oil for two weeks to see whether it is still working as a treatment, but so far each time has resumed when he begins to feel the slight twitching in his right leg, which indicates to him that he is not cured and still has the disease.

Clarence has helped to educate a number of other people with ALS in his approach to living with ALS using coconut oil and magnesium chloride and was featured in a follow-up story to Steve's and my story in early 2013 on *The 700 Club* (www.cbn.com/tv/2079485277001. A man with Parkinson's who improved dramatically using a mixture of coconut oil and MCT oil (such as in Fuel for Thought) is also featured on this video.

Some others who have held ALS at bay using coconut oil and other nutrition-based strategies are featured on the website www.alswinners.com.

I'm Still Walking!

E-mail received from another man with ALS on March 24, 2012: "I'm still walking because of *you*!. . . . I had my annual EMG on March 6, and the doctor said the test result is the same as last years. So apparently the coconut oil and magnesium chloride do work!"

Winning the Fight

Vince Tedone, a retired orthopedic surgeon living in Tampa, has taken an intensive approach to treating his daughter Deanna's ALS that is now known as the Deanna Protocol. This protocol includes coconut oil consumption and massage, as well as alpha-ketoglutarate (discussed in Chapter 4), L-arginine, CoQ10, gamma-aminobutyric acid (GABA), glutathione, nicotinamide adenine dinucleotide (NADH), and other supplements designed to improve ATP production in mitochondria, prevent glutamate toxicity (an excitatory neurotransmitter that is not metabolized normally and accumulates in ALS), and provide antioxidant effects. Deanna has had minimal worsening over more than three years with this approach.

Dr. Tedone's foundation, called Winning the Fight, is funding clinical studies on the use of the Deanna Protocol versus ketogenic and control diets in animal models with ALS at the University of

South Florida, which are already showing promising results (Ari, 2014). More information on the Deanna Protocol and these studies is available at www.winningthefight.net.

Multiple Sclerosis

Multiple sclerosis (MS) is another mysterious neurodegenerative disease that is common in younger adults between the ages of twenty and forty. The symptoms may be mild to severely disabling, sometimes with periods of remission where symptoms lessen but then flare-up again, often when the person has an infection. According to the National Institute of Neurologic Disorders and Stroke, an estimated 250,000 to 350,000 people in the United States are affected. It is unusual to die from MS and most people with this disease live a normal lifespan. MS is thought, but not proven, to be an autoimmune disease that is possibly triggered by a viral infection in which one's own antibodies inexplicably attack healthy tissues, causing inflammation and resulting in loss of myelin (the protective cover around nerve fibers), and also of nerve bodies in the brain, spinal cord, and optic nerve. The Epstein-Barr virus that causes mononucleosis has been implicated as a possible trigger, since people who had this infection as teens or young adults are more likely to develop MS.

MS: AN ATTACK ON THE NERVES

The myelin is affected in a spotty manner, analogous to squirrels chewing on a telephone line resulting in static, and so symptoms may not seem to add up and make sense at first. The most common early symptoms of MS may include problems with eye pain, double vision or blurred vision; weakness, stiffness and/or spasms of some muscles; numbness and tingling anywhere on the body; clumsiness due to balance issues; dizziness; problems with bladder control or a sudden urge to urinate. Many people go on to develop problems with mental and or physical fatigue, bipolar disease, and depression or euphoria, and problems with concentration, decision-making, planning, and prioritizing.

Like Alzheimer's disease, other dementias, and Parkinson's disease, people with MS have decreased glucose uptake in areas throughout the brain on fluorodeoxyglucose (FDG)-PET scans (Bakshi, 1998). In one study, 40 percent of people with MS had insulin resistance compared to 21 percent of the control group, and people with insulin resistance were more likely to suffer from greater disability than those without the condition (Oliveira, 2014). Also, people who have the ApoE4 gene (a major genetic risk factor for Alzheimer's) appear to be more likely to develop gray matter atrophy (shrinkage) and to develop this problem sooner on average (Horakova, 2010).

There is no cure for MS and only a handful of medications that may slow the progression in the relapsing-remitting form of the disease in the early stages, such as beta interferons, glatiramer acetate (Copaxone), and dimethyl fumarate (Tecfidera), among others. People with MS tend to have periods with sudden worsening of the disease, called "attacks." Treatments aimed at lessening the effects of these attacks include corticosteroids, plasmapheresis (plasma exchange), and medications to treat symptoms, such as muscle relaxants coupled with physical therapy.

Another approach to dealing with MS is outlined in the book by Terry Wahls, M.D., with Eve Adamson titled *The Wahls Protocol: How I Beat Progressive MS Using Paleo Principles and Functional Medicine* (2014). This protocol is mostly a dietary approach reflecting Dr. Wahls's research, initially to treat herself, and now many others. Wahls found that when she went from taking supplements to getting these same nutrients directly from the right foods, which included three cups each day of leafy green vegetables (collards, kale, spinach, etc.), sulfur-rich vegetables (asparagus, broccoli, Brussels sprouts, cabbage, etc.), and other brightly colored vegetables, she improved over a matter of months. She improved so much that she went from spending most of her time in a wheelchair to walking and even riding her bicycle again in marathons. The principles in this book are applicable to many other diseases that share the commonalities of brain inflammation and mitochondrial dysfunction.

Her new "Wahls Plus Protocol," outlined in this 2014 book, includes coconut oil (at least four to six tablespoons or about one and two-thirds cups of undiluted coconut milk per day, or a combination of the two) to raise ketone levels and provide the mitochondria with an alternative fuel to increase production of ATP; she also recommends cutting sugar intake. There are numerous testimonials in her book from people with MS who have had positive results using her protocol, including the Wahls Plus Protocol. Wahls says in her book that this is the diet she now follows herself, consuming 500 to 700 calories per day as coconut oil and/or coconut milk in addition to a variety of specific types of vegetables and moderate protein. She has a clinical trial currently underway in her patients using this ketogenic approach and is studying its impact on patients' quality of life, thinking, fatigue level, and walking ability.

A Cloud Has Lifted

E-mail sent by a young man with multiple sclerosis on September 6, 2012: "I am forty-one years old, male, and was diagnosed with relapsing-remitting multiple sclerosis in 2002. [Relapsing-remitting MS is the most common form of MS.] After four months of taking both the coconut and MCT oils, I've noticed that a thick cloud has been lifted off, as I can use my short-term memorization and I can use my mind to figure tasks in my head before I can physically perform them (do them). My mathematical formulas (numbers, math) can now be performed in my mind first."

Holding Stable

Shortly after Steve improved while taking coconut oil in 2008, I began to tell coworkers. One of them brought her sister who has MS to talk with me. She had been advised by a nutritionist in Germany nine years earlier to include coconut oil daily as a healthy fat in her diet (among other advice), and she remained quite stable during that whole time and, so far, for the years thereafter.

REPORTS OF IMPROVEMENT IN OTHER DISORDERS

In addition to the disorders discussed in Part Two, I have received reports of improvements in people with many other types of disorders who are taking coconut and/or MCT oil, including dozens with dementia not otherwise specified, mild cognitive or other memory impairment, bipolar disease, corticobasal dementia, diabetes, Down syndrome, dystonia, epilepsy, Huntington's disease, posterior cortical atrophy, and traumatic brain injury. Several people have also reported cognitive improvement in their pets.

## PART THREE

The Science

12

Diabetes of the Brain

In healthy people who have plenty of food available and who consume the typical high-carb diet, the brain uses glucose to provide nearly 100 percent of its fuel. In Alzheimer's disease, over a number of years, more and more brain cells have difficulty taking up glucose and, if no alternative fuel is provided, these important cells can malfunction and eventually die. As this problem spreads through certain areas of the brain and large numbers of brain cells are affected, symptoms begin to appear, and this process eventually results in severe cognitive and physical impairments. To be clear, in Alzheimer's disease, there are unaffected areas of the brain that use glucose normally, so glucose continues to be an important source of fuel for the brain, especially in the early to moderate stages of the disease. The problem lies in the areas that are not able to take up glucose normally.

More specifically, in Alzheimer's disease, there is insulin deficiency and insulin resistance in the brain, in essence, a type of diabetes of the brain. Insulin is required to get glucose into cells. In this chapter we will focus on this particular aspect of Alzheimer's disease, since the dietary intervention we are discussing—the use of ketones as alternative fuel to the brain—may bypass the problem of getting glucose into brain cells, a mechanism that is defective in Alzheimer's disease. Further complicating the problem with insulin, in Alzheimer's, there are deficiencies of enzymes and glucose transporters and other important substances that are also required along with insulin to get glucose into the brain, then into the neurons, and, once there, to metabolize the glucose so that it can ultimately be converted to ATP. As pointed out earlier, ATP is the final energy molecule that is needed for cells to carry out their functions. Simply put, if glucose cannot get into the cell, the cell will not be able to carry out its normal functions and may eventually die unless an alternative fuel is provided.

FORMS OF DIABETES

Diabetes (more technically, diabetes mellitus, literally "sugar diabetes") is a group of diseases in which a deficiency of insulin and/or a resistance to insulin causes glucose to build up in the blood rather than to be transported inside cells. In general, diabetes becomes more common as we age. It affects about 3.7 percent of people between the ages of twenty and forty-four, and gradually increases to nearly 27 percent in those sixty-five or older. Also, about half the U.S. population, ages sixty-five and older, have prediabetes, a condition in which glucose levels are elevated but not quite to the levels of those seen in diabetes. Therefore, more than three-quarters of the people in this age group either have diabetes or are at high risk of developing diabetes.

People with diabetes often develop other chronic conditions. It is the leading cause of kidney failure, representing about 44 percent of cases, and is also the leading cause of new cases of blindness in people between the ages of twenty and seventy-four. In addition, people with diabetes are at greater than normal risk of developing high blood pressure, heart disease, and stroke, as well as nerve damage, such as impaired sensation or pain in the extremities, skin breakdown, and difficulty with wound healing. The brain is affected as well: people with diabetes are much more likely to develop dementia than non-diabetics (Akomolafe, 2006; Pasquier, 2006).

Type 1 Diabetes

In type 1 diabetes, the pancreas fails to make insulin in response to the presence of glucose and, as a result, the glucose builds up in the blood, unable to get into the cells; this is called insulin deficiency. Without this basic fuel, the cells cannot continue to function, and when enough cells malfunction, the various organs of the body shut down.

Type 1 diabetes can develop suddenly. With this form of diabetes, the person may become acutely ill, even slipping into a coma, as the blood sugar rises and the blood becomes acidotic (too acid). In this situation, the fat cells begin to release extremely large quantities of fatty acids, which are then converted in the liver to ketones. As the ketone levels become extraordinarily high (many times higher than the levels that can be reached by consuming large amounts of coconut oil or MCT oil), a condition known as diabetic ketoacidosis develops, and the affected person will quickly die unless insulin is administered or carbohydrate is severely restricted or both. Before insulin was available as a treatment, on-and-off fasting or very high-fat, low-carb diets were sometimes utilized, but for the majority of people, death occurred within a year of onset of the disease despite these efforts.

About 3 million people in the United States have type 1 diabetes. Most cases under age ten are type 1, thus in the past this form of diabetes was called "juvenile-onset diabetes."

Type 2 Diabetes

In type 2 diabetes, the pancreas is able to make insulin but may have trouble making enough to handle the amount of glucose in the blood. Also, in some people with type 2 diabetes, certain cells do not respond normally to insulin; some of the insulin receptors may be defective or may not be on the surface of the cell membrane where they belong. In these cases, it takes higher levels of insulin to have the same effect of getting glucose into cells. Certain medications and other agents may also interfere with insulin receptors. As a result, glucose may be unable to get into the cell in sufficient amounts; this is called insulin resistance. Eventually, when the energy in the cell is depleted, the cell may go dormant or die.

Type 2 diabetes was formerly known as "adult-onset" diabetes, but it is becoming much more common in younger people, representing about one-third of cases in ten- to nineteen-year-olds. About one in five people over age sixty-five in the United States have type 2 diabetes, and there are about nine people with type 2 diabetes for each person with type 1 diabetes. It is possible to prevent type 2 diabetes and even to put it into remission by adhering to a diet that is relatively low in carbohydrates and that avoids an excess of simple sugars (like refined sugar, refined white flour, and high-fructose corn syrup), which tend to spike insulin levels. The book titled *The Art and Science of Low Carbohydrate Living* by Jeff Volek, Ph.D., and Stephen Phinney, M.D., contains an excellent and thorough discussion of the research supporting this strategy in people who are "carbohydrate intolerant," representing about three-quarters of our population. The authors suggest that keeping carbohydrate intake under 75 grams per day could keep type 2 diabetes at bay, and staying at 60 grams or below could result in ketosis in most people. Chapter 2 tackles this type of carbohydrate-limited diet.

The effects of insulin go well beyond simply letting glucose into cells. When insulin is elevated, which happens whenever carbohydrates are consumed, insulin causes fat to be stored in fat cells and reduces the use of fat as a source of energy, effectively keeping fat where it is in the fat cells. This at least partly explains why it is so easy for many type 2 diabetics with chronically elevated insulin levels to gain weight and so difficult for them to lose weight. Insulin also causes glucose to be stored in the form of glycogen in the muscles and liver. The more carbohydrates you eat, especially in the form of simple sugars, the higher your blood sugar level will go, and the higher your insulin level will rise in response. In people with insulin resistance, the constant elevation of insulin levels due to a continuously high intake of carbohydrates may interfere seriously with efforts to lose weight. A weight-loss strategy employing a low-fat, high-carbohydrate diet as is commonly recommended, even with a significant restriction of calories, would likely be much less effective at reducing body fat than a low-carb, higher-fat diet. It seems counterintuitive given the decades of national dietary policy recommendations, but look at where these policies have gotten us!

Insulin is not bad when it stays within the normal range. To the contrary, it is critical to the operation of the human body, including the brain. In addition to the functions mentioned above, insulin also affects the activity of numerous enzymes, causes the walls of arteries to relax, and enhances cell growth and survival. These are just some of the more important effects of insulin, and there are many more. It is easy then to understand that there are many health ramifications if our bodies have a problem with making insulin or with using insulin normally because the receptors are no longer responsive to insulin. Keeping insulin at normal levels, by paying close attention to the types and quantity of carbohydrates that are eaten, is key to avoiding insulin resistance.

Type 3 Diabetes (Diabetes of the Brain)

People with mild cognitive impairment, Alzheimer's disease, or other conditions that involve insulin resistance and decreased glucose uptake into the brain and other nerve cells should think of themselves as diabetic when planning their diet, even if they do not have type 1 or type 2 diabetes, and here is why.

In 2005, the term "type 3 diabetes" to describe Alzheimer's disease was coined by Suzanne de la Monte, M.D., Jack R. Wands, M.D., and their associates at Brown University in Rhode Island.

They are not the first to consider the problem of energy in the brain. In fact, as early as 1970, German physician and researcher Siegfried Hoyer found that there were decreased levels of glucose and lower metabolic rates in the brains of some people with dementia (Hoyer, 1970). Dr. Hoyer has continued to study this problem and has published numerous papers on the subject. Many other researchers have worked on various aspects of this problem since then. De la Monte's group learned that the brain makes its own insulin when they studied the brains of people with Alzheimer's disease who did not have type 1 or type 2 diabetes. They found that there was a deficiency of insulin and also insulin resistance in these brains, with features that overlap with both type 1 and type 2 diabetes elsewhere in the body (Steen, 2005). In addition, they learned that other factors involved in making and using insulin are reduced, that all the signaling pathways in the use of energy are abnormal, and that the functioning of mitochondria in the brain (the energy factories within cells) is abnormal as well.

De la Monte's group further learned, when they looked at the brains of people who had died at various stages of Alzheimer's disease and who, once again, did not have type 1 or type 2 diabetes, that this process (loss of insulin and death of affected neurons) begins early in the disease and worsens with each stage, until it is severe and occurs throughout the brain in the late stages of the disease. They have recommended that treatments for type 1 and type 2 diabetes might also help people with type 3 diabetes (de la Monte, 2008). A pilot study of intranasal insulin (given by way of the nose) showed some promise (Craft, 2012). And, in a larger study of sixty people with early-stage Alzheimer's or mild cognitive impairment, the nineteen people who received the full 40-unit dose of long-acting insulin intranasally, compared to the placebo or the lower-dose groups, showed improvement when their results were combined as a group in memory testing but not in daily functioning or executive functioning (the ability to organize and carry out tasks) testing.

However, when the results were looked at with regard to genetic types, those who were positive for the ApoE4 gene improved and those who did not carry that gene actually worsened (Claxton, 2014).

WHY IS ALL OF THIS SO IMPORTANT?

Under normal conditions, glucose is the primary fuel for our cells, including the cells of the brain, and insulin is required to allow glucose to enter our cells. Within the cell, glucose enters into a sequence of chemical reactions, which ultimately leads to the production of ATP, the final energy molecule that allows our cells to carry out their various functions. In Alzheimer's, or type 3 diabetes, as the abilities to make and use insulin, and the transport and normal use of glucose gradually become defective in the brain, brain cells malfunction and die off.

Human beings have something on the order of 100 billion nerve cells in the brain and 100 trillion synapses or connections between these cells—mind-boggling in every sense of the word! Early in the course of the disease, for ten to twenty years and possibly longer, the brain can compensate for the loss of cells and synapses, but eventually too many connections are lost and too many cells are malfunctioning or already dead, and problems such as memory loss and poor judgment begin to emerge.

One test that bears this out is the FDG-PET scan, which looks at glucose uptake in the brain. People who are known to be at risk for Alzheimer's disease by virtue of their family history may have decreased glucose uptake in the brain already in their twenties (Reiman, 2004). A 2014 report demonstrates that even young healthy infants at risk of developing late-onset Alzheimer's by virtue of carrying the ApoE4 gene already have differences in areas of the brain affected by the disease as observed on MRI scans, compared to healthy non-carriers (Dean, 2014). Specifically, the infants had lower white matter myelin water fraction (a measure of myelin content) and lower gray matter volume. The authors of the report state in their conclusion that these findings raise new questions about the role of the ApoE4 gene in normal development, in the predisposition to Alzheimer's disease, and the extent to which these brain differences might be targeted with preventive strategies. Hopefully, these infants will be followed closely over time to help determine what, if any, effects these differences in brain structure will have on them over time.

The problem of getting glucose into the brain goes beyond the problem of insulin deficiency and insulin resistance in the brain. In 1994, researchers showed that in Alzheimer's disease there are also deficiencies of two important glucose transporters: GLUT-1, which carries glucose across the membranes of the cells that make up the blood brain barrier, and GLUT-3, which carries glucose across the cell membranes of neurons (Simpson, 1994). Not only that, but it has also been known for decades that in Alzheimer's, there is a deficiency of pyruvate dehydrogenase, an enzyme in the pathway that ultimately converts glucose, with many steps between, to ATP (Hoyer, 1988). So, getting glucose into the brain and using it effectively in the brain in Alzheimer's disease is a very fundamental problem. Providing an alternative fuel to the brain and brain cells could, therefore, potentially bypass these problems.

Ketones can provide about two-thirds of the brain's energy needs during prolonged starvation and could fit the bill. It is very likely that insulin resistance plays a significant role in other forms of dementias, in Parkinson's and other neurodegenerative diseases, and even in autism, bipolar disease, and schizophrenia; each of which may show decreased glucose uptake into the brain when evaluated with an MRI. Ketones could provide relief for some people with these disorders as well.

13

Ketones as an Alternative Fuel for the Brain

Even though glucose is the brain's primary fuel, in a pinch it can easily switch to using other fuels as long as they are available. One situation in which this would occur is during a period of starvation, common in the lives of our ancestors and, sadly, even in our world today. For those of us on a typical American convenience-food diet, when we fast overnight while we sleep, virtually 100 percent of the brain's energy needs are provided by glucose and the level of ketones is negligible the next morning. However, during longer periods of starvation or intentional fasting, there is only enough glucose stored in our bodies to last about forty-eight hours, and then we must turn to other mechanisms for getting fuel to our cells. We can tap into muscle, which releases glutamine and alanine, two amino acids that are then converted primarily in the liver and kidneys to glucose, in a process called gluconeogenesis. But if muscle were our only source of fuel, we would be in big trouble since we could only expect to survive another fourteen days or so, as the muscle was gradually depleted and weakened to the point where it could no longer support our breathing.

Fortunately, human beings also have stores of fat to tap into during periods of starvation. Basically, as long as you have access to water, the fatter you are, the longer you will likely live if you cannot get food—as much as sixty days or longer—although many would not consider that a great reason to carry excess weight, given the potential negative health effects of doing so. As the body depletes its stores of glucose, fat cells release fatty acids, which the skeletal and cardiac muscle can readily use as fuel in place of glucose. But these fatty acids do not easily cross the blood-brain barrier and the brain requires a huge amount of fuel to carry on.

KETONES TO THE RESCUE

The average adult brain weighs about three pounds. Although the brain represents only 2 percent of the body's total weight, it uses roughly 20 percent of the calories we need each day to carry out basic physiological and biochemical functions; for an infant or child who has a proportionately larger brain, the brain consumes as much as 40 to 50 percent of the daily calorie requirement. So where does so much fuel come from to keep the brain alive and functioning during periods of starvation, since there is limited glucose available and fat does not easily make its way into the brain?

Some of the fatty acids released from fat cells are taken up by the liver where they are oxidized and broken down into smaller units, and some are converted to ketones, also referred to as ketone bodies, relatively small molecules that easily cross the blood-brain barrier. The presence of ketones in the circulation actually increases blood flow to the brain by as much as 39 percent (Hasselbalch, 1996). Once in the brain's circulation, ketones are rapidly taken up by the brain cells for use as fuel; this occurs regardless of whether glucose is available.

Unlike glucose, ketones do not need insulin to make their way into the cell, and they do not need as many enzymes in the complex chemical pathway that leads to the manufacture of ATP (see Figures 13.1 and 13.2). As starvation continues, over ten to twenty days, ketones continue to rise and then level off at the point where they can steadily provide as much as two-thirds of the energy needs of the brain. As long as the body continues to have stored fat, it will keep producing ketones and the cells will have enough fuel to continue operating.

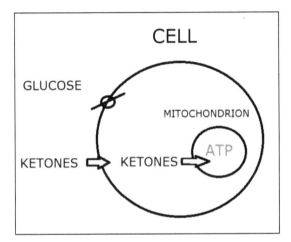

FIGURE 13.1. Simple graphic of glucose, insulin-resistance, and ketones. When there is insulin resistance in the brain, glucose does not enter the cell normally, but ketones can potentially bypass this problem and enter the pathway to make ATP, since they enter the brain cells and mitochondria by a different mechanism.

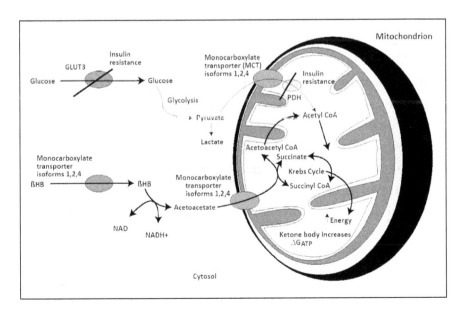

FIGURE 13.2: More complex graphic of glucose, insulin-resistance, and ketones.

Until 1967, ketones were widely believed by scientists to be just a dangerous byproduct of fat metabolism because of their association with diabetic ketoacidosis. As touched on in Chapter 12, ketone levels become extraordinarily high and coma ensues in this very abnormal situation in which there is also an absence of insulin and an extremely elevated blood glucose level. Unfortunately, many doctors today still cling to the notion that ketones are bad in every circumstance, apparently unaware of their beneficial effects at much lower levels and the crucial role they play in protecting the brain during starvation—much less the role they have played in the very survival of our species over the eons of human existence.

The fact that ketones provide the primary alternative fuel for the brain during starvation was first reported in 1967 in the article "Brain Metabolism During Fasting" in the *Journal of Clinical Investigation* by George Cahill, Jr., M.D., Oliver E. Owen, M.D., and their associates (Owen, 1967). This first case report was of an obese nurse who wanted to lose weight and volunteered to fast for forty-one days, receiving only water, salt tablets, and vitamins. The researchers took blood samples from lines placed in blood vessels around her brain and her liver to measure various metabolites, and found that her brain had survived this lengthy period of starvation by greatly increasing the use of ketones and reducing the use of glucose. Two-thirds of the fuel used by her brain was provided by beta-hydroxybutyrate and acetoacetate: two ketones produced by the breakdown of fatty acids in the liver (see Figure 13.3 on page 239 and Figure 13.4 on page 240). They also learned that glucose levels drop after about three days of starvation, along with a similar drop in insulin levels.

In a later experiment, Dr. Cahill and his associates fasted three obese college-age men until their beta-hydroxybutyrate levels were high and then gave them a dose of insulin to drive their glucose to very low levels (Cahill, 1980). Normally, without the availability of ketones, such low levels of glucose would be expected to cause

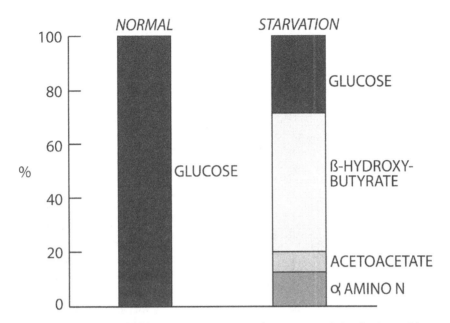

FIGURE 13.3. During an overnight fast nearly 100% of the fuel used by the brain is glucose. After a prolonged period of starvation as much as two-thirds of the energy supply to the brain comes from the ketones beta-hydroxybutyrate and acetoacetate.

serious symptoms, including confusion, difficulty thinking and speaking, weakness, poor coordination, paleness, sweating, rapid heartbeat, and even seizures, loss of consciousness, or coma. In this daring experiment, the men experienced none of these symptoms; the high level of ketones protected their brains from the potentially dire consequences of hypoglycemia (low blood sugar).

Other studies have confirmed this neuroprotective effect of ketones in the face of low blood glucose, including a study of MCT oil in type 1 diabetics (Page, 2009). In this study, type 1 diabetics who were prone to repeated attacks of hypoglycemia were given MCT oil on one occasion and a placebo on another, and then were given insulin to intentionally cause hypoglycemia. The diabetics were tested before and after the doses, which were given on two separate days, and examiners did not know which substance they

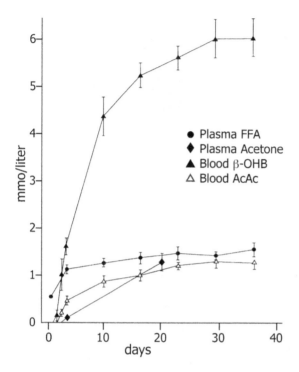

FIGURE 13.4. During starvation the ketones beta-hydroxybutyrate and acetoacetate both increase, but beta-hydroxybutyrate increases substantially more than acetoacetate over time.

received. Results showed that their memory and cognition were preserved when they received MCT oil before the insulin was given, but deteriorated when they received the placebo.

Within the past three decades, scientists have learned that the fetus is already able to produce ketones midway through the pregnancy (if not sooner), and that newborns who are exclusively breastfed will begin to produce ketones during the first twelve hours of life and use ketones to provide 25 percent of their total energy needs (Bougneres, 1986). Any first-time breastfeeding mother can tell you that there is not much volume of breast milk during the first thirty-six hours of life. So, it is for good reason that human babies are chubby when compared to other mammals, since our proportionately much larger brains require many more calories to survive. Here again, ketones come to the rescue to provide an alternative fuel for the brain to supplement the relatively meager supply of glucose available to the newborn. Glucose stores in the liver of the newborn can be used up in a matter of an hour or less compared to forty-eight hours in an adult. An interesting discussion of the importance of ketones to the fetus and newborn can be found in the book by Stephen C. Cunnane, Ph.D., titled *Survival of the Fattest: The Key to Human Brain Evolution* (2005).

OTHERS STRATEGIES TO PRODUCE KETONES

In Chapter 2, we discussed several dietary strategies for consuming MCT oil and coconut oil to raise ketone levels and make them available to the brain. Sadly, some people have reported that they or their loved one cannot seem to tolerate even a small amount of coconut or MCT oil. So, what other strategies are available to raise ketones?

Even though starvation and intentional fasting are efficient ways to produce ketones, such measures are obviously impractical for someone with Alzheimer's or some other neurodegenerative disease, and certainly not as a long-term strategy for anyone. How then can one continue to eat and produce ketones at the same time? Actually, there are several ways that we will discuss in this section.

When the body has elevated levels of ketones, it is considered to be in a state of "ketosis." Ketosis can be mild, moderate, marked, or extreme depending on the levels of ketones. Most people are familiar with the term ketosis in relation to the Atkins and South Beach diets, in which carbohydrates are restricted and ketones rise to relatively mild levels as a result of the breakdown of fat. These are variations of the classic ketogenic diet.

Classic Ketogenic Diet

The story of the effect of ketones in treating disease begins at least 2,500 years ago. There are historical references to fasting as a treatment for epilepsy and seizures as prescribed by Hippocrates, by Jesus in the New Testament (Matthew 17:14-21), and again in the Christian literature of the Middle Ages. In the 1920s, the use of prolonged periods of fasting was revived to successfully treat epilepsy. In 1921, R. M. Wilder, M.D., reported in a brief article in the *Mayo Clinic Bulletin,* titled "The Effects of Ketonemia on the Course of Epilepsy," that the ketone bodies acetone, acetoacetate, and beta-hydroxybutyrate appear not only in the urine of people in diabetic ketoacidosis but also in the urine of normal people who are starving. Not only that, but ketones appear in the urine of people who consume "a diet that contains too low a proportion of carbohydrate and too high a proportion of fat." And so, the classic "ketogenic diet" as a treatment for disease was born more than ninety years ago.

In the classic ketogenic diet, roughly 80 percent of calories come from fat and the other 20 percent come from a combination of protein and carbohydrates. Protein is limited because some of it can be converted in the liver to glucose by a process mentioned earlier called gluconeogenesis, but is high enough to allow for adequate growth in a child or to maintain muscle and other lean body mass in an adult. Ratios of fat, protein, and carbohydrates are strictly calculated and each portion of food is measured to the gram to maintain high levels of ketones, comparable to those that occur during starvation. The reward for these efforts is complete elimination of seizures in about one in four people and reduction of the number of seizures in many more.

Sadly, when antiepileptic drugs began to appear in the mid-twentieth century and were found to control seizures in most, but not all, cases, the ketogenic diet, which was used mainly for children at that time, was largely forgotten for decades, and the families of people who did not respond to these drugs believed there was no other alternative. The ketogenic diet was offered as a treatment for children in only a few places, such as Johns Hopkins Hospital, where children with multi-drug-resistant epilepsy to this day are initiated on the ketogenic diet while the family is educated in its use. Some children are able to go off the diet and continue seizure-free after just two years. More recently some adults are successfully using the ketogenic diet to control their seizures. In addition, there are a number of rare enzyme defects resulting in seizures, serious developmental delays, or both that may respond to treatment with the ketogenic diet. A listing of these can be found in a consensus report published in *Epilepsia* in 2009 (Kossoff, 2009) and also in Appendix 1.

Many physicians think the ketogenic diet is unpalatable and too difficult to adhere to, so they do not recommend, and may even discourage, the use of the diet for even their most difficult epilepsy patients. Some of these children and adults have hundreds of seizures per day and their families are unaware of the diet as a potential treatment because their doctor does not advise them of it. The families of children who have benefitted, and adults who are successfully controlling their epilepsy by adhering to the diet, would argue that the diet can be done for the long haul, can be palatable, and is a life- and brain-saver.

Thanks to the efforts of two parents of children with severe epilepsy, who stopped having nearly constant seizures within days of starting the diet, there has been a revival of the ketogenic diet worldwide and an explosion in research demonstrating its effectiveness. Around 1992, Jim Abrahams, a Hollywood director whose infant son suffered 100 or more seizures per day until he was placed on the ketogenic diet, founded the Charlie Foundation (www.charlie foundation.org). His son Charlie is now in his twenties, graduated from college, and is doing very well. He was able to resume a normal diet after seven years on the ketogenic diet with no further seizures.

Emma Williams, who learned of the ketogenic diet through Jim's efforts, founded Matthew's Friends in the United Kingdom (www.matthewsfriends.org). She asked doctors to help her put her son Matthew on the diet for six years before one finally agreed, and his seizures stopped within days. She has said that she often wonders how much less long-term brain damage could have been avoided if his doctors had agreed to let him try the diet much sooner.

Together, Jim and Emma have reached hundreds of thousands of families dealing with epilepsy, and have inspired and supported the establishment of ketogenic diet centers around the world. Their foundations alternate sponsoring a symposium on the status of the ketogenic diet in treatment of epilepsy and other diseases every two years, with some presentations geared toward professionals and others for families. The last three conferences were expanded to include discussions of ketogenic diets in Alzheimer's disease, autism, cancer, GLUT-1 transporter deficiency and other enzyme deficiencies causing seizures, and traumatic brain injury. The next conference will be held in Banff, Canada, in the fall of 2016.

In recent years, some less stringent variations of the classic high-fat ketogenic diet have been developed, and research has shown that many patients with epilepsy improve with these diets as well. Three such diets are the modified MCT oil–ketogenic diet, in which 60 percent of the calories in the diet come from MCT oil; the low-glycemic index diet, which avoids simple sugars; and the modified Atkins diet, which limits protein compared to the original Atkins diet in which protein was unlimited.

As mentioned previously, a pilot study using a classic ketogenic diet in people with Parkinson's disease resulted in considerable improvement on average (VanItallie, 2005). One man with Parkinson's has reported to me that he had some improvement while taking frequent doses of coconut oil, but that there was a lot of fluctuation, especially in his tremor. He feels that he has had more consistent improvement with less fluctuation while on a strict ketogenic diet. This approach could be a viable option for some people who don't see results with coconut or MCT oil.

Exercise and Ketosis

The body can go into a state of mild temporary ketosis from exercise. Known for years as the Courtice-Douglas effect, and named for scientists who studied it in the 1930s, post-exercise ketosis was first discovered by G. Forssner in 1909, who found that levels of ketones always increased in his urine after a brisk, thirty-six-minute, four-kilometer (two-and-one-half mile) walk before breakfast. Subsequent studies found that mild ketosis can be sustained for nine hours or longer after vigorous exercise, but that ketosis does not occur following exercise if a high-carbohydrate meal is eaten first. Perhaps this effect of post-exercise ketosis at least partly explains the purported beneficial effect of exercise in the prevention of dementia. In addition, recent studies have shown that vigorous exercise, such as forced stationary bicycle riding, can reduce symptoms of Parkinson's disease as well (Ridgel, 2009). Once again, could ketosis at least partly explain this phenomenon?

Ketone Ester and Other Ketone-Containing Substances

Yet another way to increase ketones through diet is to consume them in the form of esters or other ketone-containing substances, such as ketone triacylglycerides and ketone mineral salts. It has been shown with ketone-PET scanning that the blood level of ketones is directly proportional to the amount of ketones that enter the brain; in other words, if the ketone level is high in the blood, there will be more ketones available for the brain to use as fuel (Cunnane, 2011). The great advantage to ketone esters is that a single dose can raise ketone levels to 5 mmol/L or even higher, which could provide as much as two-thirds of the energy requirement of the brain, and if consumed on a regular basis could potentially halt or even reverse the process of Alzheimer's disease. Another product called ketone triacylglyceride combines three molecules of the ketone beta-hydroxybutyrate with glycerol to form a structure much like a triglyceride. The ketone acetoacetate has been formulated into an ester product called acetoacetate diester and is also used in another product combined with minerals such as sodium, potassium, calcium, and magnesium to form ketone mineral salts. These products are made for research purposes at present to study for use in various medical conditions and for improving physiologic performance, and are ultimately expected to become available to the public as foods, medical foods, or drugs once they are recognized as such by the FDA.

As mentioned previously, it was first reported by Dr. Cahill and his associates in 1967 that ketones are used by the brain as an alternative fuel during starvation when glucose stores are depleted. The study of ketones, what they do, and how they might be useful in the treatment of disease found a home in the early 1990s in the lab of Richard L. Veech, M.D., at the NIH. Dr. Veech received his medical degree from Harvard and completed a research fellowship at the NIH, followed by a three-year stint where he honed his skills as a biochemist at Oxford University in England in the lab of Nobel Prize winner Hans Krebs (for his discovery of the citric acid cycle). In their first published studies of ketone effects, Dr. Veech and his associates found that rat hearts pump harder using less oxygen when ketones are in the mix and that ketones are able to duplicate nearly all the acute effects of insulin. In other words, ketones are a type of super fuel that is even more efficient than glucose at producing energy within the mitochondria of the cell, and that can substitute for both glucose and insulin during starvation when glucose is not readily available and insulin levels are therefore low (Kashiwaya, 1994).

Confirming and expanding on this with further studies, and in association with Kieran Clarke, Ph.D., at Oxford University, Dr. Veech and his associates began to develop a ketone ester. Ketones are acidic and, in order for them to be taken orally, need to be attached to another molecule that the stomach lining and intestinal tract will tolerate. One way, as in Dr. Veech's formulation, is to attach the ketone beta-hydroxybutyrate to an alcohol, such as 1,3-butanediol, to form what is known as a ketone ester. Butanediol is recognized as safe by the FDA for use as an additive to foods and is commonly used as a humectant (an agent that helps retain moisture). In a somewhat delayed reaction, butanediol is also converted to ketones after it is absorbed from the gastrointestinal tract and broken apart from the ketone. Combining the ketone with butanediol can help prolong the elevation of the ketone level.

In 2000, Dr. Veech and his associates reported in a landmark study that when neurons in one set of cultures were subjected to a substance known to cause Alzheimer's disease, if the ketone beta-hydroxybutyrate was added to the mix at levels comparable to those that occur during starvation, many more neurons survived than if the ketone was not added. Furthermore, the same held true for neurons in cultures that were exposed to a substance that causes Parkinson's disease (Kashiwaya, 2000). This study further confirmed the neuroprotective effects of ketones and the potential usefulness of the ketone ester to treat Alzheimer's, Parkinson's, and potentially a plethora of diseases in which there is a problem of glucose uptake into cells. A series of hypothesis papers were published shortly thereafter discussing the potential of the ketone ester to treat disease, authored by three important pioneers and long-time associates in the area of ketone research: Dr. Veech, Dr. Cahill, and Dr. VanItallie (Cahill, 2003; VanItallie, 2003; Veech, 2001, 2004).

By 2006, Dr. Veech's group hit upon a successful formulation of ketone ester with the scientific name (R)-3-hydroxybutyl (R)-3-hydroxybutyrate, which has subsequently shown no significant adverse effects during toxicity testing in fifty-four healthy adults, as reported in 2012 (Clarke, 2012), and has since received GRAS status from the FDA for use in healthy adults.

Studies of the effects of the ketone ester in mice continued as well. And, in 2012, results were published of a groundbreaking study by Dr. Veech and his group using a mouse model with Alzheimer's, which showed a decrease in both plaques and tangles in the brain, as well as reduced anxiety and subtle improvements in learning and memory, in the mice that were fed the ketone ester (Kashiwaya, 2013). Another article reported that feeding mice the ketone ester increased the number of mitochondria in the cells of brown fat, which did not occur when using a high-fat ketogenic diet to raise ketones to the same level (Srivastava, 2012).

A great advantage to using the ketone ester is that considerably higher levels of ketones can be easily achieved without any other changes to the diet compared to the much lower levels obtained with using MCT oil or coconut oil or a low-carb diet. Table 13.1 compares ketone levels that can be reached with various ketone-producing strategies. (By comparison, levels in diabetic ketoacidosis reach 25 mmol/L.)

TABLE 13.1. STRATEGIES TO INCREASE KETONE LEVELS	
STRATEGY	**KETONE LEVELS**
Coconut oil/MCT oil*	0.3–0.5 mmol/L
Vigorous exercise	0.3–0.5 mmol/L
Ketone mineral salts*	0.5–2.0 mmol/L
Starvation	2–5 mmol/L
Classic ketogenic diet	2–5 mmol/L
Ketone esters*	2–5 mmol/L or higher
Diabetic ketoacidosis	25 mmol/L

*Note: Will increase ketone levels without restricting carbohydrate in diet and will also lower blood glucose level.

A promising report of a single case of a man (my husband, Steve) with early-onset Alzheimer's disease using Dr. Veech's ketone ester documents significant improvement in cognition and ability to perform activities of daily living that were sustained for a twenty-month period. I hope that this case report will trigger funding for, at the very least, a pilot study of the ketone ester in Alzheimer's disease (Newport, 2015).

So, why isn't this ketone ester on the market yet? When produced in a relatively small lab, ketone ester is very expensive to make, and sufficient funding has not come forth from the NIH or another source to mass-produce the ester—even though it could be accomplished at considerably lower cost when made on a larger scale. Nor has funding come through so that human clinical trials can be undertaken to study its use in disease. In order to be studied as an investigational new drug, the FDA requires $10 million, and this does not include the cost of making the ketone ester or recruiting and testing patients, which would require many millions more.

At present, the U.S. government spends less than $500 million per year on Alzheimer's research. This is a fraction of what is spent to study cancer and HIV, in spite of the estimated 5.2 million people suffering from the disease and the more than 500,000 people dying each year from complications of it. Ketone ester may be the most promising of treatments, but it is vying with many other entities for these meager research dollars. Still, there is some good news: a technique has been developed in Dr. Veech's lab to produce the ester very inexpensively when made in a large lab with fermentation capability. Hopefully, the planets will align in the near future for those who so desperately need the ketone ester with adequate funding, the right company to make it, and centers to test it in people with Alzheimer's, Parkinson's, and other diseases.

Meanwhile, interest is growing in developing and studying ketone esters and other means of raising ketones for a variety of diseases. At the University of South Florida in Tampa, animal research is ongoing under the direction of Dominic D'Agostino, Ph.D., to look at the effects of these strategies on cancer (see next), Alzheimer's, ALS, wound healing, oxygen toxicity, epilepsy, status epilepticus, and traumatic brain injury.

Beyond Alzheimer's: Ketogenic Diet and Cancer

A recent development in the use of the ketogenic diet to treat disease is to control the growth of cancer. The driving force behind this is Thomas Seyfried, Ph.D., the premier researcher of ketogenic diets for brain cancer, a professor of biology at Boston College, and the author of *Cancer as a Metabolic Disease* (2012), which explains the history and concepts behind this strategy. His initial work in this area was with glioblastoma, an aggressive brain cancer (Seyfried, 2014), but he and his collaborators are studying this approach in other types of cancer as well; several human clinical trials are now underway.

Most cancer cells thrive on sugar and metabolize it in a primitive way, since the mitochondria are defective. This defect was discovered more than eighty years by Nobel Prize winner Otto Warburg but, much like the ketogenic diet for epilepsy, was put on the back burner until Dr. Seyfried and others began to intensely investigate this concept once again. The defect in mitochondria also prevents the cancer cells from using ketones effectively as an alternative fuel, whereas normal cells of the brain and other organs can continue to use ketones in place of glucose. By maintaining a strict ketogenic diet and restricting caloric intake to keep the blood glucose as low as possible, tumor cells begin to die off and the cancerous tumor shrinks; in addition, metastases (the spread of cancer cells) shrink and die off as well. The diet could potentially be used alone or in conjunction with standard treatments for cancer.

Dr. Seyfried's collaborator at the University of South Florida, Dr. D'Agostino, is researching additional strategies for further reducing the blood sugar while optimizing ketone levels to protect the brain in order to treat cancer. Dozens of human volunteers with various types of cancer are having positive results. More information about this can be found on Dr. D'Agostino's website at www.ketonutrition.org and his blog at www.ketonutrition.blog spot.com. Additional helpful information can be found in a book written by Ellen Davis titled *Fight Cancer with a Ketogenic Diet* (2014) and another by Elaine Cantin called *The Cantin Ketogenic Diet for Cancer, Type 1 Diabetes, and Other Ailments* (2012).

Help for the Caregivers Is Long Overdue

ighty-seven percent of caregivers are relatives of the person with dementia. So many people trying to care for their loved ones must watch them slowly and painfully deteriorate. At first they forget little things like where they have placed their wallet or keys. Ultimately, they forget how to do the simplest things they have done for a lifetime, such as sitting down and standing up. Worst of all, they fail to recognize the people who love and care for them, the child they gave birth to or the spouse they married many years earlier. The problem of dementia goes way beyond forgetfulness. The brain is so complex that, when affected by a disease such as Alzheimer's, the bizarre and inexplicable occur, and the nightmare only gets worse with each stage of the disease. Just what I mean here is difficult to explain to an outsider. Alzheimer's caregivers know exactly what I am talking about.

Support and education for family caregivers is sparse compared to the number of people dealing with the problem. Most caregivers must develop the patience and skills needed by trial and error to help their loved ones get in and out of bed, bathe and clothe themselves, assist with toileting or deal with incontinence (no small task), and ensure they receive adequate nutrition, which in the later stages involves hand-feeding often for hours every day. As the disease progresses, caregivers must often deal with serious neuropsychiatric and behavioral issues, such as anxiety, agitation, wandering, depression, sleeplessness, aggression, even screaming, biting, and kicking in some people. Some of these behaviors go on for hours on end and throughout the night (since sleep disturbances are very common), an extremely stressful and exhausting situation for those who are dealing with this at home.

In the later stages of the disease, people with Alzheimer's cannot be left unattended and eventually they become completely unable to care for themselves. Caregivers who are fighting this battle alone often become severely isolated, exhausted, sleep-deprived, and depressed. Family members who are not living in the home with the Alzheimer's loved one often do not fully appreciate the extreme amount of time and attention required, and how desperately the primary caregiver needs a break from the routine that other family members could provide to help them get through this difficult situation. Family members should not assume the caregiver will ask for help if needed or that they will not know what to do if they do step in to help. By coming to the caregiver's rescue on a regular basis, the rescuer will quickly learn, just as the primary caregiver did, how to tend to the loved one's needs. Some couples have no family or friends to help them and it is hard to comprehend how one person alone can deal day in and day out with caring for a spouse with Alzheimer's at home.

Care of people with Alzheimer's disease and other dementias imposes a major financial burden on the average family, since only a few hours a week of home health care are generally covered by Medicare and private insurance. In addition, the bulk of charges for assisted living, averaging $42,600 per year, are not usually covered by private insurance or Medicare until the person requires skilled nursing care—unless one was fortunate enough to have purchased expensive long-term care insurance before symptoms appeared. Medicaid will only pay for care in facilities after the person's assets, and much of the spouse's assets, have been depleted. The amount of assets the spouse is allowed to keep varies from state to state, but there is a federal minimum and maximum.

Alzheimer's disease is not being recognized as the medical condition that it is, a complication of a form of diabetes, so that the very expensive but necessary care is not worthy of coverage by private health insurance, Medicaid, or Medicare. Treatment of other complications of diabetes, such as renal failure, eye disease, and poor circulation, resulting in slow wound healing and sometimes amputation are covered by private insurance and Medicare. Why, then, after a lifetime of carrying insurance and paying into Medicare through employment, must a person deplete his or her own assets to provide medically necessary care for a spouse with Alzheimer's or some other dementia? To add insult to injury, it is very common for the caregiver to have to cut back and then give up working altogether in order to provide what eventually becomes 24/7 care. The payback for years of caregiving, whether accomplished at home or in assisted living, is too often the loss of one's own future financial stability.

Hopefully, as more and more evidence accumulates that Alzheimer's disease is a form of diabetes of the brain, a medical condition akin to diabetes type 1 and type 2, the bulk of the financial burden will transfer from the family to Medicare and private insurance. A new definition of what constitutes medically necessary care needs to emerge for people with Alzheimer's, other dementias, and neurodegenerative diseases.

This picture of Alzheimer's disease is bleak, but this is just the reality that too many millions are currently dealing with.

Many good books on caregiving are available and some recommendations are listed in the Resources section at the end of this book. For far too many people, caregiving is learned by trial and error, as there is not nearly enough support and education for the millions dealing with the disease. Many of us tend to find out for the first time what the symptoms of Alzheimer's are—some of them quite unanticipated—as they appear in our loved ones. Many of the things that happen at the hands of a person in even the earlier stages of Alzheimer's simply do not make sense and often present a safety risk. Advanced education of caregivers could allow for better anticipation and preparation for these problems, potentially reducing the number of tragic events that occur simply because the caregiver and other family members were unaware of what *could* occur. Other caregivers have agreed with me that words cannot begin to convey the day-to-day and minute-to-minute reality of living with someone who has Alzheimer's, coupled with the fact that such caregiving may go on for many years. The harsh reality is that, not only have the lives of the victims been hijacked, but the lives of the caregivers as well.

It would be most helpful for those who are involved in caregiver support and education to have real, extensive, firsthand experience that would bring true empathy to the job. A few years ago I attended a caregiver training series and found it disappointing that the person running the program and doing the teaching had not been a direct hands-on caregiver for a family member with Alzheimer's. He meant well, but the best he could do when people had questions was to use examples of dealing with his children. Any of us with real experience can tell you that Alzheimer's caregiving is nothing akin to caring for children. Toilet training for a 30-pound two- or three-year-old, who will soon learn, can be frustrating but is very different from trying to reteach a 200-pound, seventy-five-year-old man, who no longer recognizes what a toilet is for, fights it with all his might, and will likely have a major accident followed by a major clean-up of him and his surroundings while you are trying to get him to the bathroom. Imagine that you are his 130-pound, seventy-five-year-old wife with your own health issues, that you are undertaking this alone, and that this episode lasts an hour or longer several times a day. If you can imagine this scenario, then you will mentally step into the shoes of far too many who *are* dealing with this alone. This is just one of many nightmare scenarios caregivers deal with on a daily basis and, just when you think you are already living in a bad dream, your nightmare gets inexplicably worse. An estimated 40 percent of Alzheimer's patients are cared for at home until they pass away.

While, in my opinion, experiencing Alzheimer's caregiving should ideally be a prerequisite for teaching it, it is unrealistic to expect researchers and funders of research to have such firsthand experience, though many are genuinely motivated by such personal experience. The reality of living with Alzheimer's disease is still a big secret and this needs to change. If lawmakers could see first-hand what is going on in millions of homes in the United States and many-fold more worldwide, then perhaps the relatively meager dollars earmarked for Alzheimer's disease would greatly increase, not only to find strategies for prevention and meaningful treatment but also to educate one-on-one and provide in-home support for the caregivers. Many caregivers have no choice but to give up their day job to care for their spouse or parent with Alzheimer's; understandably, most will be happy to leave Alzheimer's in the dust when their loved one passes on. But for those who are up to it, taking on the role of education and support for the next generation of caregivers would be invaluable. The government and Alzheimer's associations should consider recruiting such people for paid positions to take on this Herculean task.

How helpful it would be to develop an extensive collection of unedited video footage of people at various stages of the disease in home and assisted-living settings, to follow individuals over the course of their disease, and to collect interviews with caregivers about what they are going through—real people dealing with this very real problem. Such a collection would be invaluable for educational purposes for those involved in research, as well as decision-making for policy and funding.

An excellent, comprehensive study of the current status of

dementia care and the plight of caregivers throughout the world is available on the Alzheimer's Disease International website at www.alz.co.uk/research/WorldAlzheimerReport2013.pdf. In this report, the authors state, "Caregiver multicomponent interventions (comprising education, training, support, and respite) maintain caregiver mood and morale, and reduce caregiver strain. This is also the only intervention that has been proven to reduce or delay transition from home into a care home. Such interventions seem to be particularly effective when applied early in the journey of care. Nevertheless, we are aware of no governments that have invested in this intervention to scale-up provision throughout the dementia care system, and hence coverage is minimal." It is time for that to change.

Fifty Conditions That May Respond to Raising Ketones

A number of conditions share the problem of decreased glucose uptake in the brain, nerves, or cells of other organs, as demonstrated by abnormal PET scans or measures of insulin resistance, and/or are associated with mitochondrial dysfunction. Many of these conditions have already been shown in small- to moderate-size clinical trials to benefit from a low-carb, high-fat, protein-sufficient ketogenic diet and others have yet to be studied. Theoretically, these conditions could also potentially benefit from treatments that elevate ketones through other methods, such as medium-chain triglycerides (coconut oil, MCT oil), ketone esters, or ketone mineral salts, which will hopefully become available to the general public soon. Elevation of ketones by diet or by any of these other methods could also potentially bring about improvement by reducing inflammation, which is a common feature of neurodegenerative diseases. It is important that treatments with various ketone-raising interventions and/or a ketogenic diet are discussed with the person's physician to determine if they are justified and would not be harmful or possibly worsen the disease.

Conditions that may respond to ketone-raising dietary interventions include:

- Age-related memory impairment
- Alcohol abuse
- Amyotrophic lateral sclerosis
- Alzheimer's disease

- Autism (many children also respond to gluten-free or carbohydrate-specific diets)
- Birth asphyxia
- Bovine spongiform encephalopathy (also known as mad cow disease)
- Cancer (strict ketogenic diet, possibly with addition of ketone esters or ketone mineral salts)
- Chronic stress
- Conditions requiring steroid use
- Corticobasal degeneration
- Creutzfeldt-Jakob disease
- Cushing's disease
- Dementia associated with Pick's disease
- Dementia of Parkinson's with frontal atrophy
- Diabetes (types 1 and 2)
- Diseases with chronic inflammation
- Down syndrome (associated Alzheimer's in middle age)
- Epilepsy (including some rare enzyme defects and specific syndromes associated with epilepsy)
- Friedreich's ataxia
- Frontal temporal lobe dementia (also called primary progressive aphasia)
- Glaucoma
- GLUT-1 deficiency syndrome
- Glycogen-storage diseases
- Huntington's disease (also called Huntington's chorea)
- Hypoglycemia of the newborn (affects about 10 percent of newborns)
- Infant of diabetic mother (IDM) syndrome
- Leigh's syndrome
- Leprechaunism (also called Donohue syndrome)
- Lewy body dementia
- Metabolic syndrome
- Mild cognitive impairment (often a precursor to Alzheimer's disease)
- Mitochondrial myopathies
- Multiple sclerosis
- Muscular dystrophy
- Myasthenia gravis
- Optic atrophy
- Optic neuropathy

- Oxygen toxicity
- Parkinson's disease (with or without dementia)
- Polycystic ovarian syndrome
- Poor wound healing
- Posterior cortical atrophy (also called Benson's syndrome)
- Prediabetes (insulin resistance)
- Progressive supranuclear palsy
- Pyruvate dehydrogenase deficiency
- Rabson-Mendenhall syndrome
- Russell-Silver syndrome
- Stroke
- Sudden lack of oxygen
- Traumatic brain injury
- Vascular dementia (often occurs along with Alzheimer's disease)

There are some rare genetic disorders in which ketone-raising dietary interventions should absolutely not be used. People with epilepsy of unknown origin should be screened for the following diseases before undertaking a ketogenic diet or using other ketone-raising interventions:

- Primary carnitine deficiency
- Carnitine palmitoyltransferase I or II deficiency
- Carnitine translocase deficiency
- Beta-oxidation defects
- Short-chain acyl-CoA dehydrogenase deficiency
- Medium-chain acyl-CoA dehydrogenase deficiency
- Long-chain acyl-CoA dehydrogenase deficiency
- Medium-chain 3-hydroxyacyl-CoA deficiency
- Long-chain 3-hydroxyacyl-CoA deficiency
- Pyruvate carboxylase deficiency
- Porphyria

Ketone esters and ketone salts have shown great promise in targeting the following rare genetic enzyme defect but not coconut oil, MCT oil, or a ketogenic diet:

• Multiple acyl-CoA dehydrogenase deficiency

Other conditions that are contraindicated for ketone-raising dietary interventions include:

• Intractable epilepsy that testing determines could be alleviated by surgery

• Non-compliant parent or caregiver

• Severe liver disease

• Allergy to coconut (for those who would use coconut oil)

Lastly, a strict ketogenic diet is contraindicated for the following condition, with the exception of coconut oil, which could be beneficial for weight gain and weight stabilization:

• Inability to maintain adequate nutrition (becoming very thin or emaciated due to poor appetite)

Possible Causes and Contributors to Alzheimer's Disease

The list of culprits that may cause or contribute to the development of Alzheimer's disease is long. Very likely there is more than one trigger that sets off the disease process. The brain does not have an obvious external outlet for ridding itself of waste products and toxins as, for example, the gastrointestinal and respiratory tracts do. Scientists are only starting to understand the mechanism that the brain uses to rid itself of cellular waste products and other debris. This mechanism appears to be dysfunctional in people with neurodegenerative diseases and begins to help explain the accumulation of waste products like beta-amyloid that are found in the brain (Nedergaard, 2012). In addition, the brain is extremely protective of what can get in and out of the blood-brain barrier, and this system is also defective in people with Alzheimer's disease. Not only that, but certain components of the immune system become weaker as we reach old age, which allows microorganisms of many types also to accumulate in the brain.

When one thinks about the sheer number of different potentially harmful chemicals that the brain is exposed to on a daily basis, it is small wonder that we are in the midst of an epidemic of neurodegenerative diseases. Our ancestors who consumed whole foods, often fresh off the tree or bush, probably wouldn't recognize much of what we are eating today. Almost certainly, Alzheimer's disease must be ultimately triggered by something coming into the brain by way of the nose or mouth.

Here are some of the known predisposing factors, possible causes, or contributing factors to the development of Alzheimer's disease:

- **Genetic predisposition:** The vast majority of people with Alzheimer's do not have a genetic predisposition for the disease. A number of different genes have been shown to carry a greater risk of developing Alzheimer's if they are in our genes. The best known of these include:

  o *Presenilin 1 and 2.* The percentage of people who carry gene mutations leading to familial Alzheimer's disease is 0.1 percent. The most common are mutations in the presenilin 1 or 2 gene that appear to increase deposition of amyloid proteins in plaques in the brain.

  o *Apolipoprotein E4 (ApoE4).* Inheriting the ApoE4 gene from one or both parents increases risk, with an even greater likelihood of developing the early-onset form of the disease if one has two copies of the gene.

  o *Down syndrome (trisomy 21).* Having an extra copy of chromosome 21 (the cause of the syndrome) carries some of the Alzheimer's-related genes. People with Down syndrome have a very high rate of developing Alzheimer's in middle age and have plaques in the brain already early in childhood.

- **Diabetes:** People with type 1 or type 2 diabetes have a higher than usual risk of developing dementia, and an even greater risk if they have also had episodes of hypoglycemia (low blood sugar) serious enough to require hospitalization. Research by R. Scott Turner, M.D., director of Georgetown University Medical Center's Memory Disorders Program, found that undiagnosed prediabetes is common in the early stages of Alzheimer's disease, suggesting that all people with Alzheimer's should be screened for diabetes. Turner discovered this when recruiting non-diabetics with Alzheimer's disease for a trial with resveratrol, a substance found in red grapes and red wine that may increase blood sugar (glucose). After performing a glucose-tolerance test on the potential candidates, he found that 43 percent had either diabetes (13 percent) or prediabetes (30 percent) and were apparently unaware of this when they applied for the clinical trial. Turner presented these findings at the Alzheimer's Association International Congress in Boston on July 14, 2013 (ADIN, 2013).

- **Traumatic brain injury:** A head injury severe enough to cause loss of consciousness increases the risk of developing dementia later in men by twofold, and with repeated concussions, as in football players and boxers, the risk is many times greater (Mortimer, 1991; Fleminger, 2003; Schwarz, 2009).

- **Chronic sleep apnea:** Sleep apnea is a condition that may lead to dementia and that can contribute to memory impairment due to repeated nightlong interruptions in breathing, which reduce oxygen flow to the brain and prevent deep sleep. This condition is often treatable, and such treatment could potentially lessen or prevent symptoms of dementia.

- **Environmental factors and lifestyle choices:** Certain substances may damage DNA and/or other structures in the cell and cell membrane and/or cause oxidative damage and inflammation, one of the hallmarks of Alzheimer's and other neurodegenerative diseases. Several of these substances include:

  ○ *Pollutants* such as air pollution, smoking of tobacco (which contains nitrosamine compounds), and chronic inhalation or skin exposure to pesticides.

  ○ *Food additives* (directly or by way of the animal's food supply), including antibiotics and hormones; nitrates, nitrites, and other preservatives; artificial sweeteners, colors, and flavorings; sugar, fructose, and high-fructose corn syrup; hydrogenated or partially hydrogenated fats with trans fats; pesticides; and nitrite-containing fertilizers and fertilizer residue in and on fruits and vegetables.

○ *Toxic metals* such as aluminum, cadmium, lead, and mercury (and even some metals like copper, iron, manganese, and zinc that are needed to carry out normal cell functions) can cause damage in excessive amounts resulting in accumulation in the brain. Taking certain supplements and multivitamin products could be more harmful than helpful in this regard and getting the natural form of vitamins and trace elements from food would be the ideal.

- **Dietary deficiencies:** Deficiencies of certain nutrients are associated with memory impairment and other symptoms of dementia, including several B vitamins such as cobalamin (B_{12}) and folic acid (although excessive folic acid may also be harmful); vitamin D; and omega-3 fatty acids, specifically docosahexaenoic acid (DHA), which is found in marine sources of omega-3 such as krill and coldwater fatty fish.

- **Excessive alcohol intake:** Alcohol in and of itself may cause damage to brain cells and, in addition, some beers and hard liquors such as scotch are still being processed with damaging nitrosamine compounds.

- **Infectious agents:** Recurrent fever blisters caused by herpes simplex virus type 1 (HSV-1) are much more common in people who carry the ApoE4 gene. A host of microorganisms have been implicated in a variety of other diseases involving the brain and nervous system, such as those that cause syphilis, influenza, polio, measles, mononucleosis, mumps, Lyme's disease, and Creutzfeldt-Jakob disease (mad cow disease).

- **Autoimmune diseases:** Overreaction of the immune system results in inflammation and destruction of important proteins in the brain that could cause or contribute to dementia. For example, in a common viral infection like HSV, the sequence of amino acids in the proteins of HSV is identical to the sequence of amino acids in portions of the tau proteins that make up the skeleton of the neuron in the axons and dendrites. It is, therefore, likely that the antibodies (immune system proteins that recognize and destroy specific substances) that attack the herpes virus would also attack the tau protein (Carter, 2011). A similar phenomenon exists with other viruses, bacteria, and fungi including *Chlamydia pneumonia* (bacteria that cause pneumonia and also found in Alzheimer's brains), *Porphyromonas gingivalis* (bacteria that cause gum disease and known risk factor for Alzheimer's), and human herpesvirus 5 (also called cytomegalovirus) and human herpesvirus 6. There are three organisms that may result in dementia or memory impairment but cognitive function may improve when treated: *Cryptococcus neoformans* (fungi that cause lung infections), *Helicobacter pylori* (bacteria that cause ulcers), and *Borrelia burgdorferi* (bacteria that cause Lyme's disease).

- **Medications:** Anticholinergic drugs block the nervous system neurotransmitter acetylcholine from attaching to receptors in the brain and may contribute to symptoms of fogginess, confusion, and memory impairment. Anticholinergics may also counter the effects of Alzheimer's medications such as Aricept and Exelon that increase availability of acetylcholine by decreasing the breakdown of the substance. Benzodiazepines, corticosteroids, and antipsychotics may cause side effects, some quite severe, that may be incorrectly attributed to worsening of the person's dementia. Statins (cholesterol-lowering medications) may cause memory impairment. In addition, many drugs and breakdown products of drugs can accumulate in the brain. Might these foreign chemicals damage surrounding brain structures directly or provoke an inflammatory immune response?

- **Anesthesia:** Anesthetics such as isoflurane (Forane) may result in cognitive impairment for days to months (or longer) following surgery.

For a more extensive discussion of how these factors may cause or contribute to the disease process, see *Alzheimer's Disease: What If There Was a Cure? The Story of Ketones.*

The Seven Stages of Alzheimer's Disease

For many the earliest symptoms of Alzheimer's disease are related to memory, but others first experience changes in behavior and personality. They have trouble organizing, they make poor decisions, they have great difficulty sleeping, and they experience visual disturbances that originate in the brain (not the eye). Depression is common, whether part of the process itself, or a result of awareness that something is desperately wrong. Many people are able to cover up the issues for a time and still function normally in social situations, but they can only hide so much from someone who lives with them every day. It is common for friends, family members outside the victim's home, and the doctor to dismiss a spouse or partner's concerns—a very frustrating situation.

The Alzheimer's Association recognizes seven stages of Alzheimer's disease, having recently added a preclinical stage in which the disease process is underway but there are no obvious symptoms. Since nearly all the newer drugs tested to date have aimed at reducing amyloid plaque in the brain and have had little or no impact on improving memory and other aspects of cognitive performance, there is a new movement toward focusing research efforts on finding treatments and strategies that may delay or prevent the onset of symptoms.

For those who are at risk, one of the current dilemmas is whether testing for Alzheimer's disease should be done. There are several sides to this issue: one view is that because there are no effective drugs to treat the disease at present, there is no point to knowing one's risk since this information may cause anxiety and depression.

A second view is that this information could allow one to become more proactive and motivated to make lifestyle choices that could result in delay or prevention of the disease. I know of many people who have had one or more family members with Alzheimer's and who suffer from anxiety and depression just knowing that they could be affected. For these people, testing could either confirm what they already suspect (that they are at higher risk) or reduce their worry (if negative) and provide great relief to learn that they are no more likely than the average person to develop the disease. Even people who carry two copies of the ApoE4 gene, one from each parent, will not necessarily acquire the disease. In these cases, knowledge can be power. It gives people the opportunity to make lifestyle changes such as quitting smoking, getting tested for and treated for sleep apnea, reducing sugar intake and eating a healthier whole-food diet, and increasing exercise. It allows people to plan their finances and to get their legal ducks in a row by drafting a will and a living will, and to put on paper whom they wish to designate as their healthcare surrogate and power of attorney. People can do things on their bucket list now rather than putting them off for another ten or twenty years while expecting they will enter the golden years in good health.

Yet, a third view is to forget testing and to make these changes anyway to reap the potential all-around health benefits.

Here is a summary of the seven stages of Alzheimer's disease as outlined by the Alzheimer's Association (with my two cents added). Keep in mind that there is considerable overlap between the stages and that an individual may not experience all signs and symptoms and may have additional problems not mentioned here.

Stage 1: No impairment (normal function). The disease process is underway but there are no obvious symptoms.

Stage 2: Very mild cognitive decline (may be normal age-related changes or earliest signs of Alzheimer's disease). The person is aware of memory lapses but symptoms of dementia are not yet detected by others. Cognitive testing is normal.

Stage 3: Mild cognitive decline (early-stage Alzheimer's disease can be diagnosed in some, but not all, individuals with these symptoms). Signs of the disease become more noticeable to others and can be detected with appropriate interviewing and testing. Some problems may include losing or misplacing valuable objects, difficulty coming up with the right word or name, trouble with planning or organizing, trouble retaining new information, and/or difficulty carrying out tasks that could be completed previously.

Stage 4: Moderate cognitive decline (mild or early-stage Alzheimer's disease). Symptoms are readily detected with appropriate interviewing and testing, and may include problems in several areas such as forgetting recent events and details of one's own past, social withdrawal, moodiness, greater difficulty carrying out complex tasks such as budgeting and paying bills, and trouble performing somewhat complex mental math. This is the point at which many people with Alzheimer's are unable to continue functioning satisfactorily in their jobs.

Stage 5: Moderately severe cognitive decline (moderate or mid-stage Alzheimer's disease). Problems with memory and thinking become much more obvious to others and may include forgetting one's own address, where one is and what day it is, and some, but not all, important details of his or her life. The person may need help with many day-to-day activities such as choosing appropriate clothing, but is usually able to eat and use the toilet without assistance. Simple mental math is now more difficult.

Stage 6: Severe cognitive decline (moderately severe or mid-stage Alzheimer's disease). Memory continues to deteriorate and the person needs assistance and/or supervision to successfully carry out most activities of daily living, such as eating and toileting, and may experience loss of control of urine and bowel movements. The person may recognize some family and friends by name but not the spouse or the caregiver at all times, and may not recognize him- or herself in a mirror. There is a high risk of wandering and sleep disturbances are common, with more confusion occurring later in the day in many people, often called "sundowning" or "sundowner's syndrome." Major changes in mood, personality, and behavior may emerge such as constant anxiety and pacing; fearfulness; hallucinations; false beliefs; repetitive behaviors such as hand wringing and picking at the skin; and violence such as biting, punching, and kicking. Some people develop physical symptoms as well, suggestive of some overlap with Parkinson's disease (tremors, slow shuffling gait, stiffness), and falls are common. It is sometimes difficult to sort out which of these behavioral and physical symptoms are a result of the disease process or the side effects of medications.

Stage 7: Very severe cognitive decline (severe or late-stage Alzheimer's disease). During the final stage, typically lasting one to three years, the person deteriorates and eventually becomes bed bound, is usually incontinent, must be fed, and relies on others for all personal care. Many people become rigid, cannot sit up unsupported or hold their head up, and can no longer smile and communicate effectively. Urinary tract infections as well as pneumonia and choking due to aspiration of food are common. Very disturbed sleep patterns may occur, with long periods of sleeplessness. Eventually, the person forgets how to chew and swallow food and will likely die due to dehydration and malnutrition, unless artificial nutrition with a tube is undertaken. It is important for people to establish a living will when they are competent to make their wishes known so that the appropriate decisions can be made by family members when this stage in the disease process arrives.

Resources

Suggested Reading

The following books are good sources of information for those who wish to explore further the topics discussed in this book.

Bowden, Jonny, and Stephen Sinatra. *The Great Cholesterol Myth: Why Lowering Cholesterol Won't Prevent Heart Disease—and the Statin-Free Plan That Will.* Beverly, MA: Fair Winds Press, 2012.

Buckley, Julie A., and Jenny McCarthy. *Healing Our Autistic Children: A Medical Plan for Restoring Your Child's Health.* New York: Palgrave MacMillan, 2010.

Buettner, Dan. *The Blue Zones.* 2nd ed. Washington, DC: National Geographic Society, 2012.

Calbom, Cherie. *The Coconut Diet.* New York: Warner Books, 2005.

_____. *The Ultimate Smoothie Book.* New York: Wellness Central/ Hachette Book Group, Inc., 2006.

Cantin, Elaine. *The Cantin Ketogenic Diet for Cancer, Type 1 Diabetes, and Other Ailments.* Williston, VT: Self-published, 2012.

Chou, Charles, with Debbie Ng. *Coconut Oil Secret Exposed.* Singapore: Smile Forever Digital Press, 2013.

Cunnane, Stephen C. *Survival of the Fattest: The Key to Human Brain Evolution.* Singapore: World Scientific Publishing Company, 2005.

Davis, Ellen. *Fight Cancer with a Ketogenic Diet.* 2nd ed. Ebook, 2014. Available from www.ketogenic-diet-resource.com/cancer-diet.html.

Davis, William. *Wheat Belly: Lose the Wheat, Lose the Weight, and Find Your Path Back to Health.* New York: Rodale Books, 2011.

Enig, Mary. *Know Your Fats*. Silver Spring, MD: Bethesda Press, 2000.

_____ and Sally Fallon. *Eat Fat, Lose Fat*. New York: Penguin Group, 2005.

_____ and _____. *Nourishing Traditions*. 2nd ed. Washington, DC: New Trends Publishing Inc., 2001.

Erasmus, Udo. *Fats That Heal, Fats That Kill*. Summertown, TN: Books Alive, 2008 (originally published in 1986).

Fife, Bruce. *Coconut Lover's Cookbook*. 4th ed. Colorado Springs, CO: Piccadilly Books, Ltd., 2010.

_____. *Coconut Oil Miracle*. 5th ed. Colorado Springs, CO: Piccadilly Books, Ltd., 2013.

_____. *Oil Pulling Therapy*. Colorado Springs, CO: Piccadilly Books, Ltd, 2008.

_____. *Stop Alzheimer's Now!* Colorado Springs, CO: Piccadilly Books, Ltd., 2011.

_____. *Stop Autism Now*. Colorado Springs, CO: Piccadilly Books, Ltd., 2011.

Fife, Bruce, and Conrado S. Dayrit. *Coconut Cures*. Colorado Springs, CO: Piccadilly Books, Ltd., 2005.

Frayne, Catherine. *Thoughts of Yesterday*. Galway, Ireland: Book Hub Publishing, 2013.

Freeman, John, Eric Kossoff, Jennifer Freeman, and Millicent Kelly. *The Ketogenic Diet*. 4th ed. New York: Demos Medical Publishing, 2007.

Graveline, Duane. *Lipitor: Thief of Memory*. Self-published, 2006.

_____. *Statin Damage Crisis*. 3rd ed. Self-published, 2012.

_____. *Statin Drugs, Side Effects*. 5th ed. Self-published, 2008.

Gursche, Siegfried. *Coconut Oil*. Summertown, TN: Books Alive, 2008.

Heimowitz, Colette. *The New Atkins Made Easy*. New York: Touchstone, 2013.

Jackson, Grace E. *Drug-Induced Dementia: A Perfect Crime*. Bloomington, IN: Author House, 2009.

Kossoff, Eric H., John M. Freeman, Zahava Turner, et al. *Ketogenic Diets*. New York: Demos Medical Publishing, 2011.

Lands, William. *Fish, Omega-3 and Human Health.* 2nd ed. Urbana, IL: AOCS Press, 2005.

LeBlanc, Gary J. *Staying Afloat in a Sea of Forgetfulness: Common Sense Caregiving.* Bloomington, IN: Xlibris Corporation, 2010.

_____. *Managing Alzheimer's and Dementia Behaviors: Common Sense Caregiving.* Parker, CO: Outskirts Press, Inc, 2012.

Lombard, Jay, and Carl Germano. *The Brain Wellness Plan.* New York: Kensington Books, 2000.

London, Jan. *Coconut Cuisine: Featuring Stevia.* Summerton, TN: Book Publishing Company, 2006.

Lord, Ethelle G. *How in the World . . . and Now What Do I Do? A Primer for Alzheimer's: 12 Major Points for Coping Better.* Ebook, 2013. Available from http://AlzheimersPrimer.com.

_____. *Alzheimer's Coaching: Taking a Systems Approach to Creating an Alzheimer's Friendly Healthcare Workforce.* Mustang, OK: Tate Publishing, 2015.

MacBean, Valerie. *Coconut Cookery.* Berkeley, CA: Frog Books, 2001.

Mace, Nancy, and Peter Rabins. *The 36-Hour Day.* New York: Time Warner Book Group, 2001.

McCully, Kilmer S. *The Heart Revolution.* New York: Perennial/Harper Collins Books, 1999.

Newport, Mary T. *Alzheimer's Disease: What If There Was a Cure? The Story of Ketones.* 2nd ed. Laguna Beach, CA: Basic Health Publications, Inc., 2013.

Nutribase. *The Nutribase Complete Book of Food Counts.* New York: Avery, 2001.

Perlmutter, David, M.D. *Grain Brain.* New York: Little, Brown and Company, 2013.

Price, Weston A. *Nutrition and Physical Degeneration.* 8th ed. La Mesa, CA: The Price-Pottenger Nutrition Foundation, 2008 (first published in 1939).

Seyfried, Thomas. *Cancer as a Metabolic Disease.* Hoboken, NJ: John Wiley & Sons, 2012.

Schopick, Julia. *Honest Medicine.* Oak Park, IL: Innovative Health Publishing, 2011.

Simopoulos, Artemis, and Jo Robinson. *The Omega Diet.* New York: Harper Collins Publishers, Inc., 1999.

Sinatra, Stephen. *The Sinatra Solution: Metabolic Cardiology.* Laguna Beach, CA: Basic Health Publications, 2008.

Snowdon, David. *Aging with Grace.* New York: Bantam Books, 2001.

Snyder, Deborah. *Keto Kid.* New York: Demos Medical Publishing, 2007.

Stoll, Andrew L. *The Omega-3 Connection.* New York: Simon & Schuster, 2001.

Tobin, Alicia, and Chris Gursche. *Keto-Genesis.* Westminster, BC: Foresight Publishing, 2015.

Vanderhaeghe, Lorna, and Karlene Karst. *Healthy Fats for Life.* 2nd ed. Toronto: John Wiley & Sons, 2004.

VanRyzin, Christine. *Alzheimer's Averted: A Path to Survival.* Appleton, WI: Elemental Basic Publishing, 2004.

Volek, Jeff, and Stephen Phinney. *The Art and Science of Low Carbohydrate Living.* Miami, FL: Beyond Obesity, LLC, 2011.

Wahls, Terry. *Minding My Mitochondria: How I Overcame Secondary Progressive Multiple Sclerosis (MS) and Got Out of My Wheelchair.* Iowa City, IA: TZ Press, 2010.

Wahls, Terry, with Eve Adamson. *The Wahls Protocol: How I Beat Progressive MS Using Paleo Principles and Functional Medicine.* New York: Penguin Publishing Group, 2014.

Westman, Eric, Jeff Volek, and Stephen Phinney. *The New Atkins for a New You.* New York: Touchstone, 2010.

Zook, Sylvia. *Eatin' After Eden.* Tucson, AZ: Wheatmark, 2008.

Audiovisual Links

Calhoun, Cecilia. "Dr. VanItallie Interview, Parts I–XI." Cognate Nutritionals, 29:35. Mar 28, 2014. Available at www.youtube.com/watch?v=3_Lsor-kWxg&list=PLQxrx8FHaqT-7C-UYqT0C5qZAc_88BXKD.

Johnson, Lorie. "Alzheimer's Doctors Taking Note of Coconut Oil." *The 700 Club*, 11:58. Jan 7, 2013. Available at www.cbn.com/cbnnews/ healthscience/2013/January/Alzheimers-Doctors-Taking-Note-of-Coconut-Oil-/?_ga=1.191072938.1240434222.1427580309.

_____. "Coconut Oil Touted as Alzheimer's Remedy" *The 700 Club*, 6:02. Jan 5, 2012. Available at www.cbn.com/cbnnews/healthscience/ 2012/January/Coconut-Oil-Touted-as-Alzheimers-Remedy/?_ga= 1.27561276.1240434222.1427580309.

Institute for Human and Machine Cognition. "Mary Newport—Medium Chain Triglycerides and Ketones: An Alternative Fuel for Alzheimer's." Public lecture held at the Institute for Human and Machine Cognition, 1:04:00. March 6, 2013. Available at www.youtube.com/watch?v= feyydeMFWy4&list=PLedklXpZ22n5uhTRKnZBp9m-0n WEnhs3k.

Lightburn, Ken. "Alzheimer's—Must Watch—Dr. Mary Newport— Coconut Oil MTCs." Six-segment interview with Ken Lightburn, 55:29. Oct 11, 2009. Available at www.youtube.com/watch?v=_9INyTTXfR0.

Resource Organizations

The following is a list of organizations and medical websites that can provide additional information on all aspects of Alzheimer's disease and other neurologic conditions.

Alzheimer's Association: www.alz.org

Alzheimer's Disease Cooperative Study: www.adcs.org

Alzheimer's Disease International: www.alz.co.uk

Alzheimer's Family Organization: www.alzheimersfamily.org

National Institute on Aging, Alzheimer's Disease Education and Referral Center: www.nia.nih.gov/alzheimers

National Institute of Neurologic Disorders and Stroke: www.ninds. nih.gov

National Institutes of Health, Clinical Trials Registry: www.clinical trials.gov

National Parkinson Foundation: www.parkinson.org

Apps, Forums, Blogs, Foundations, and Message Boards

ALS Forums: www.alsforums.com

Alzheimer's Association message board: www.alz.org/living_with_alzheimers_message_boards_lwa.asp

Alzheimer's Reading Room: www.alzheimersreadingroom.com

Alzheimer's Research Forum: www.alzforum.org

The Alzheimer's Spouse: www.thealzheimerspouse.com

CareGiving App: www.caregivingapp.com

Dementia and Alzheimer's Weekly: www.alzheimersweekly.com

Dr. Newport's website: www.coconutketones.com

Dr. Newport's blog: www.coconutketones.blogspot.com

International Caregivers Association: www.internationalcaregiversassociation.com

Jimmy Moore's Livin' La Vida Low-Carb: www.livinlavidalowcarb.com

KetoNutrition—Metabolic Strategies for Neurodegenerative Diseases and Cancer: www.ketonutrition.org and www.ketonutrition.blogspot.com

Michael J. Fox Foundation for Parkinson's Research: www.michaeljfoxfoundation.org

Parkinson's Research Foundation: www.parkinsonhope.org

Remi Savioz GLUT-1 Deficiency Syndrome (RSG1) Foundation: www.remisglut1foundation.com

Wahls Protocol: www.terrywahls.com

Winning the Fight (Against ALS): www.winningthefight.net

Sources for Coconut Oil and MCT Oil

The following websites offer an array of coconut oil and MCT oil products.

Alpha Health Products: www.alphahealth.ca

Amazon.com: www.amazon.com

Barlean's Organic Oils: www.barleans.com

Cheap Vitamins: www.cheapvitamins.com

Coconut Oil Online: www.coconutoil-online.com

Coeurisma Coconut Oil and Chocolate Coconut Oil: www.coeurisma.com

Cognate Nutritionals: www.fuelforthought.co

Costco: www.costco.com

Earth Balance: www.earthbalancenatural.com

Memory Pharmacy: www.memorypharmacy.com

Nature's Approved: www.naturesapproved.com

Nisshin Oillio: www.nisshin-oillio.com/english/company/index.shtml

Niulife: www.niulife.com.au

Nutiva: http://nutiva.com

Parrillo Performance: www.parrillo.com

Sam's Club: www.samsclub.com

Spectrum: www.spectrumorganics.com

Swanson Health Products: www.swansonvitamins.com

Tropical Traditions: www.tropicaltraditions.com

True Protein: www.trueprotein.com

Wilderness Family Naturals: www.wildernessfamilynaturals.com

Coconut Oil Information

Coconut Research Center: www.coconutresearchcenter.org

Ketogenic Diet Information and Support

The Charlie Foundation: www.charliefoundation.org

KetoNutrition—Metabolic Strategies for Neurodegenerative Diseases and Cancer: www.ketonutrition.org and www.ketonutrition.blogspot.com

Ketopet: www.ketopet.com

Matthew's Friends: www.matthewsfriends.org

RSG1 Foundation: www.remisglut1foundation.com

References and
Related Articles

Preface

Aisen PS, LJ Thal, SH Ferris, et al. Rofecoxib in patients with mild cognitive impairment: further analyses of data from a randomized double-blind trial. *Curr Alzheimer Res* Vol 5 (2008): 73-82.

Introduction

Ari C, AM Poff, HE Held, et al. Metabolic therapy with Deanna Protocol supplementation delays disease progression and extends survival in amyotropic lateral sclerosis (ALS) mouse model. *PLoS One* Vol 9, No 7 (2014): 1–9.

Brownlow ML, L Benner, D D'Agostino, et al. Ketogenic diet improves motor performance but not cognition in two mouse models of Alzheimer's pathology. *PLoS One* Vol 8, No 9 (2013): 1–10.

Chiu S, C Chen, H Cline. Insulin receptor signaling regulates synapse number, dendritic plasticity, and circuit function in vivo. *Neuron* Vol 58, No 5 (2008): 708–719.

D'Agostino DP, R Pilla, HE Held, et al. Therapeutic ketosis with ketone ester delays central nervous system oxygen toxicity seizures in rats. *Am J Physiol Regul Integr Comp Physiol* Vol 304 (2013): R829–R836.

Edwards C, J Canfield, N Copes, et al. D-beta-hydroxybutyrate extends lifespan in *C. elegans. Aging* Vol 6, No 8 (2014): 1–24.

Nafar F and KM Mearow. Coconut oil attenuates the effects of amyloid-beta on cortical neurons in vitro. *J Alzheimer's Dis* Vol 39 (2014): 233–237.

Poff AM, C Ari, P Arnold, et al. Ketone supplementation decreases tumor cell viability and prolongs survival of mice with metastatic cancer. *Int J Cancer* Vol 135, No 7 (2014): 1711–1720.

Seyfried TN, J Marsh, P Mukherjee, et al. Could metabolic therapy become a viable alternative to the standard of care for managing glioblastoma? *Hematology and Oncology Review* Vol 10, No 1 (2014): 13–20.

Uemura E, HW Greenlaw. Insulin regulates neuronal glucose uptake by promoting translocation of glucose transporter GLUT3. *Exp Neurol* Vol 198, No 1 (2006): 48–53.

Chapter 2

Astarita G, K-M Jung, NC Berchtold, et al. Deficient liver biosynthesis of docosahexaenoic acid correlates with cognitive impairment in Alzheimer's disease. *PLoS One* Vol 5, No 9 (2010): 1–8.

Basu S, P Yoffe, N Hills et al. The relationship of sugar to population-level diabetes prevalence: an econometric analysis of repeated cross-sectional data. *PLoS One* Vol 8 (2013): e57873.

Crane PK, R Walker, RA Hubbard, et al. Glucose levels and risk of dementia. *N Engl J Med* Vol 369, No 6 (2013): 540–548.

Dashti HM, NS Al-Zaid, TC Mathew, et al. Long-term effects of ketogenic diet in obese subjects with high cholesterol level. *Mol Cell Biochem* Vol 286 (2006): 1–9.

De la Monte SM, A Neusner, J Chu, et al. Epidemiological trends strongly suggest exposures as etiologic agents in the pathogenesis of sporadic Alzheimer's disease, diabetes mellitus, and non-alcoholic steatohepatitis. *J Alzheimers Dis* Vol 17 (2009): 519–529.

De la Monte SM, M Tong. Mechanisms of ceramide-mediated neurodegeneration. *J Alzheimers Dis* Vol 16, No 4 (2009): 704–714.

Food and Drug Administration. FDA takes step to further reduce *trans* fats in processed foods. Press release, Nov. 7, 2013. Available at www.fda.gov/newsevents/newsroom/pressannouncements/ucm373939.

Gross LS, L Li, ES Ford, et al. Increased consumption of refined carbohydrates and the epidemic of type 2 diabetes in the United States: an ecological assessment, *Am J Clin Nutr* Vol 79 (2004): 774–779.

Guyenet S. By 2606 the U.S. diet will be 100 percent sugar. *Whole Health Source: Nutrition and Health Science* www.wholehealthsource.blogspot.com, February 18, 2012.

Institute of Medicine. *Dietary Reference Intakes for Energy, Carbohydrate, Fiber, Fat, Fatty Acids, Cholesterol, Protein, and Amino Acids.* Washington, DC: National Academies Press, 2005.

Lakhan SE, A Kirchgessner. The emerging role of dietary fructose in obesity and cognitive decline. *Nutrition Journal* Vol 12 (2013): 114.

Martinez-Lapiscina EH, P Clavero, E Toledo, et al. Mediterranean diet improves cognition. *J Neurol Neurosurg Psychiatry* Vol 84, No 12 (2013): 1318–1325.

Sinatra ST, BB Teter, J Bowden, et al. The saturated fat, cholesterol, and statin controversy: A commentary. *JACN* Vol 33, No 1 (2014):79–88.

U.S. Department of Agriculture. *Dietary Guidelines for Americans, 2010.* 7th ed. Washington, DC: U.S. Government Printing Office, 2010. Available at http://health.gov/dietaryguidelines/dga2010/dietaryguidelines2010.pdf.

Volek JS, SD Phinney, CE Forsythe, et al. Carbohydrate restriction has a more favorable impact on the metabolic syndrome than a low fat diet. *Lipids* Vol 44 (2009): 297–309.

Chapter 3

Castellano A, S Nugent, S Tremblay, et al. In contrast to lower brain glucose uptake, brain ketone uptake is unchanged in mild Alzheimer's disease: A dual tracer PET study comparing 18F-FDG and 11C-acetoacetate. *CTAD*, San Diego, Nov 15, 2013.

Choi CU, HS Seo, EM Lee, et al. Statins do not decrease small, dense low-density lipoprotein. *Tex Heart Inst J* Vol 37, No 4 (2010): 421–428.

Chowdhury R, S Warnakula, S Kunutsor, et al. Association of dietary, circulating, and supplement fatty acids with coronary risk. *Ann Intern Med* Vol 160 (2014): 398–406.

Costantini LC, LJ Barr, JL Vogel, et al. Hypometabolism as a therapeutic target in Alzheimer's disease. *BMC Neurosci* Vol 9, Suppl 2 (2008): S16.

Cunnane S, S Nugent, M Roy, et al. Brain fuel metabolism, aging, and Alzheimer's disease. *Nutrition* Vol 27, No 1 (2011): 3–20.

Evans MA, BA Golomb. Statin-associated adverse cognitive effects: survey results from 171 patients. *Pharmacotherapy* Vol 27, No 7 (2009): 800–811.

Golomb BA. Implications of statin adverse effects in the elderly. *Expert Opin Drug Saf* Vol 4, No 3 (2005): 389–397.

Golomb BA, MA Evans. Statin adverse effects: a review of the literature and evidence for a mitochondrial mechanism. *Am J Cardiovasc Drugs* Vol 8, No 6 (2008): 373–418.

Mauger J, AH Lichtenstein, LM Ausman, et al. Effect of different forms of dietary hydrogenated fats on LDL particle size. *Am J Clin Nutr* Vol 78 No 3 (2003): 370–375.

Mulder M, R Ravid, DF Swaab, et al. Reduced levels of cholesterol, phospholipids, and fatty acids in cerebrospinal fluid of Alzheimer disease patients are not related to apolipoprotein E4. *Alzheimer Dis Assoc Disord* Vol 12 (1998): 198–203.

Poff AM, C Ari, P Arnold, et al. Ketone supplementation decreases tumor cell viability and prolongs survival of mice with metastatic cancer. *Int J Cancer* Vol 135, No 7 (2014): 1711–1720.

Poplawski M, JW Mastaitis, F Isoda, et al. Reversal of diabetic nephropathy by a ketogenic diet. *PLoS One* Vol 6, No 4 (2011): 1–9.

Reger MA, ST Henderson, C Hale, et al. Effects of Beta-hydroxybutyrate on cognition in memory-impaired adults. *Neurobiol Aging* Vol 25 (2004): 311–314.

Ren J, I Dimitrov, AD Sherry, et al. Composition of adipose tissue and marrow fat in humans. *J Lipid Res* Vol 49, No 9 (2008): 2055–2062.

Schatz IJ, K Masaki, K Yano, et al. Cholesterol and all-cause mortality in elderly people from the Honolulu Heart Program: a cohort study. *Lancet* Vol 358 (2001): 351–355.

Seneff S, G Wainwright, L Mascitelli. Nutrition and Alzheimer's disease: the detrimental role of a high-carbohydrate diet. *Eur J Intern Med* Vol 22, No 2 (2011): 134–140.

Siri PW, RM Krauss. Influence of dietary carbohydrate and fat on LDL and HDL particle distributions. *Curr Atheroscler Rep* Vol 7, No 6 (2005): 455–459.

Studzinski CM, WA MacKay, TL Beckett, et al. Induction of ketosis may improve mitochondrial function and decrease steady-state amyloid-beta precursor protein (APP) levels in the aged dog. *Brain Res* Vol. 1226 (2008): 209–217.

Taha AY, ST Henderson, WM Burnham. Dietary enrichment with medium-chain triglycerides (AC-1203) elevates polyunsaturated fatty acids in the parietal cortex of aged dogs: implication for treating age-related cognitive decline. *Neurochem Res* Vol 34, No 9 (2009): 1619–1625.

Toft-Petersen AP, HH Tilsted, J Aarphe, et al. Small dense LDL particles—a predictor of coronary artery disease evaluated by invasive and CT-based techniques: a case-control study. *Lipids Health Dis* Vol 10, No 21 (2011): 1–7.

Chapter 4

Ari C, AM Poff, HE Held, et al. Metabolic therapy with Deanna Protocol supplementation delays disease progression and extends survival in amyotrophic lateral sclerosis (ALS) mouse model. *PLoS One* Vol 9, No 7 (2014): 1–9.

Auestad N, RA Korsak, JW Morrow, et al. Fatty acid oxidation and ketogenesis by astrocytes in primary culture. *J Neurochem* Vol 56, No 4 (1991): 1376–1386.

Bergen SS, SA Hashim, TB VanItallie. Hyperketonemia induced in man by medium-chain triglyceride. *Diabetes* Vol 15, No 10 (1966): 723–725.

Bitman J, L Wood, M Hamosh, et al. Comparison of the lipid composition of breast milk from mothers of term and preterm infants. *Am J Clin Nutr* Vol 38 (1983): 300–312.

Cabré E, E Domènech. Impact of environmental and dietary factors on the course of imflammatory bowel disease. *World J Gastroenterol* Vol 18, No 29 (2012): 3814–3822.

Castellano CA, S Nugent, N Paquet, et al. Lower brain 18F-fluorodeoxyglucose uptake but normal 11C-acetoacetate metabolism in mild Alzheimer's disease dementia. *J Alzheimers Dis* Vol 43 (2015): 1343–1353.

Castellano CA, S Nugent, S Tremblay, et al. In contrast to lower brain glucose uptake, brain ketone uptake is unchanged in mild Alzheimer's disease: A dual tracer PET study comparing 18F-FDG and 11C-acetoacetate. *CTAD*, San Diego, Nov 15, 2013.

Costantini LC, LJ Barr, JL Vogel, et al. Hypometabolism as a therapeutic target in Alzheimer's disease. *BMC Neurosci* Vol 9, Suppl 2 (2008): S16.

Cunnane S, S Nugent, M Roy, et al. Brain fuel metabolism, aging, and Alzheimer's disease. *Nutrition* Vol 27, No 1 (2011): 3–20.

Field T, M Diego, M Hernandez-Reif. Preterm infant massage therapy research: a review. *Infant Behav Dev* Vol 33, No 2 (2010): 115–124.

Henderson ST. Ketone bodies as a therapeutic for Alzheimer's disease. *Journal of the American Society for Experimental NeuroTherapeutics* Vol 5 (2008): 470–480.

Isaacs CE, KS Kim, and H Thormar. Inactivation of enveloped viruses in human bodily fluids by purified lipids. *Ann NY Acad Sci* Vol 724 (1994): 457–464.

Isaacs CE, RE Litov, H Thormar. Antimicrobial activity of lipids added to human milk, infant formula, and bovine milk. *J Nutr Biochem* Vol 6, No 7 (1995): 362–366.

Maynard SD, J Gelblum. Retrospective case studies of the efficacy of caprylic triglyceride in mild-to-moderate Alzheimer's disease. *Neuropsychiatr Dis Treat* Vol 9 (2013): 1629–1635.

Maynard SD, J Gelblum. Retrospective cohort study of the efficacy of caprylic triglyceride in patients with mild-to-moderate Alzheimer's disease. *Neuropsychiatr Dis Treat* Vol 9 (2013): 1619–1627.

Page KA, A Williamson, N Yu, et al. Medium-chain fatty acids improve cognitive function in intensively treated type 1 diabetic patients and support in vitro synaptic transmission during acute hypoglycemia. *Diabetes* Vol 58, No 5 (2009): 1237–1244.

Reger MA, ST Henderson, C Hale, et al. Effects of beta-hydroxybutyrate on cognition in memory-impaired adults. *Neurobiol Aging* Vol 25 (2004): 311–314.

Ren J, I Dimitrov, AD Sherry, et al. Composition of adipose tissue and marrow fat in humans. *J Lipid Res* Vol 49, No 9 (2008): 2055–2062.

Shea JC, MD Bishop, EM Parker, et al. An enteral therapy containing medium-chain triglycerides and hydrolyzed peptides reduces postprandial pain associated with chronic pancreatitis. *Pancreatology* Vol 3, No 1 (2003): 36–40.

Sucher K. Medium-chain triglycerides: a review of their enteral use in clinical nutrition. *Nutr Clin Prac* Vol 44 (1986): 146–150.

Sulkers EJ, HN Lafeber, HJ Degenhart, et al. Comparison of two preterm formulas with or without addition of medium-chain triglycerides (MCTs): II: effects on mineral balance. *J Pediatri Gastroenterol Nutr* Vol 15, No 1 (1992): 42–47.

Svensson M, JW Eriksson. Insulin resistance in diabetic nephropathy—cause or consequence? *Diabetes Metab Res Rev* Vol 22, No 5 (2006): 401–410.

Tantibhehyangkul P, SA Hashim. Medium-chain triglyceride feeding in premature infants: Effects on fat and nitrogen absorption. *Pediatrics* Vol 55 (1975): 359–370.

Turner N, K Hariharan, J TidAng, et al. Enhancement of muscle mitochondrial oxidative capacity and alterations in insulin action are lipid species dependent: potent tissue-specific effects of medium-chain fatty acids. *Diabetes* Vol 48 (2009): 2547–2554.

Wozniak MA, RF Itzhaki. Antiviral agents in Alzheimer's disease: hope for the future? *Ther Adv Neurol Disord* Vol 3 (2010): 141–152.

Chapter 7

Alzheimer's Association. 2014 Alzheimer's Disease Facts and Figures. *Alzheimer's & Dementia* Vol 10, No 2 (2014). Also available from www.alz.org/downloads/Facts_Figures_2014.pdf.

Doody RS, R Raman, M Farlow, et al. A phase 3 trial of semagacestat for treatment of Alzheimer's disease. *N Engl J Med* Vol 369, No 4 (2013): 341–350.

James BD, SE Leurgans, LE Hebert, et al. Contribution of Alzheimer disease to mortality in the United States. *Neurology* Vol 82 (2014): 1045–1050.

Chapter 8: Non-Alzheimer's Dementias

National Institute on Aging. *Lewy Body Dementia: Information for Patients, Families and Professionals*. National Institutes of Health: Bethesda, MD, 2013. Also, available from www.nia.nih.gov/sites/default/files/lewybodydementia-no_drop_shadow_13dec23.pdf.

Chapter 9: Parkinson's Disease

Aviles-Olmos I, P Limousin, A Lees, et al. Parkinson's disease, insulin resistance and novel agents of neuroprotection. *Brain* Vol 136, No 2 (2013): 374–384.

VanItallie TB, C Nonas, A Di Rocco, et al. Treatment of Parkinson disease with diet-induced hyperketonemia: a feasibility study. *Neurology* Vol 64 (2005): 728–730.

Chapter 10: ALS

Ari C, AM Poff, HE Held, et al. Metabolic therapy with Deanna Protocol supplementation delays disease progression and extends survival in amyotrophic lateral sclerosis (ALS) mouse model. *PLoS One* Vol 9, No 7 (2014): 1–9.

Field T, M Diego, M Hernandez-Reif. Preterm infant massage therapy research: a review. *Infant Behav Dev* Vol 33, No 2 (2010): 115–124.

Turner N, K Hariharan, J TidAng, et al. Enhancement of muscle mitochondrial oxidative capacity and alterations in insulin action are lipid species dependent: potent tissue-specific effects of medium-chain fatty acids. *Diabetes* Vol 48 (2009): 2547–2554.

Van Laere K, A Vanhee, J Verschueren, et al. Value of [18]fluorodeoxyglucose-positron-emission tomography in amyotrophic lateral sclerosis: a prospective study. [1]KU Leuven, Nuclear Medicine and Molecular Imaging, University Hospital Leuven, Leuven, Belgium

[2]KU Leuven, Department of Neurology, University Hospital Leuven, Leuven, Belgium

[3]KU Leuven, Department of Neurosciences, Experimental Neurology, and Leuven Research Institute for Neuroscience and Disease (LIND), Leuven, Belgium

[4]VIB, Vesalius Research Center, Laboratory of Neurobiology, Leuven, Belgium

JAMA Neurol Vol. 71, No. 5 (2014): 553–561.

Chapter 11

Bakshi R, RS Miletich, PR Kinkel, et al. High-resolution fluorodeoxyglucose positron emission tomography shows both global and regional cerebral hypometabolism in multiple sclerosis. *J Neuroimaging* Vol 8, No 4 (1998): 228–234.

Horakova D, M Kyr, E Havrdova, et al. Apolipoprotein E [e]4-positive multiple sclerosis patients develop more gray-matter and whole-brain atrophy: a 15-year disease history model based on a 4-year longitudinal study. *Folia Biol (Praha)* Vol 56, No 6 (2010): 242–251.

National Institute of Neurological Disorders and Stroke. NINDS multiple sclerosis information page. National Institutes of Health, May 21, 2014. Also available from www.ninds.nih.gov/disorders/multiple_sclerosis/multiple_sclerosis.htm.

Oliveira SR, ANC Simao, AP Kaullar, et al. Disability in patients with multiple sclerosis: Influence of insulin resistance, adiposity, and oxidative stress. *Nutrition* Vol 30, No 3 (2014): 268–273.

Chapter 12

Claxton A, LD Baker, A Hanson, et al. Long-acting intranasal insulin Detemir improves cognition for adults with mild cognitive impairment or early-stage Alzheimer's disease dementia. *J Alzheimers Dis* 2014 Nov 5 [Epub ahead of print].

Craft S, LD Baker, TJ Montine, et al. Intranasal insulin therapy for Alzheimer disease and amnestic mild cognitive impairment: a pilot clinical trial. *Arch Neurolog* Vol 69, No 1 (2012): 29–38.

De la Monte SM, JR Wands. Alzheimer's disease is type 3 diabetes—evidence reviewed. *J Diabetes Sci Technol* Vol 2, No 6 (2008): 1101–1113.

Dean III DC, BA Jerskey, K Chen, et al. Brain differences in infants at differential genetic risk for late-onset Alzheimer's: A cross-sectional imaging study. *JAMA Neurol* Vol 71, No 1 (2014): 11–22.

Hoyer S, K Oesterreich, O Wagner. Glucose metabolism as the site of the primary abnormality in early-onset dementia of Alzheimer type? *J Neurol* Vol 5, No 3 (1988): 143–148.

Hoyer S. Brain metabolism and the incidence of cerebral perfusion disorders in organic psychoses. *Deutsche Zeitschrift für Nervenheilkunde* Vol 197, No 5 (1970): 242–292.

Reiman EM, K Chen, GE Alexander, et al. Functional brain abnormalities in young adults at genetic risk for late-onset Alzheimer's dementia. *PNAS* Vol 101, No 1 (2004): 284–289.

Simpson IA, KR Shundu, T Davies-Hill, et al. Decreased concentrations of GLUT1 and GLUT3 glucose transporters in the brains of patients with Alzheimer's disease. *Ann Neurolog* Vol 35 (1994): 546–¬551.

Steen E, BM Terry, EJ Rivera, et al. Impaired insulin and insulin-like growth factor expression and signaling mechanisms in Alzheimer's disease: Is this type 3 diabetes? *J Alzheimers Dis* Vol 7, No 1 (2005): 63–80.

Chapter 13

Bougneres PF, C Lemmel, P Ferre, et al. Ketone body transport in the human neonate and infant. *J Clin Invest* Vol 77, No 1 (1986): 42–48.

Cahill Jr, GF, TT Aoki. Alternate fuel utilization by brain. In *Cerebral Metabolism and Neural Function*. Edited by JV Passonneau, RA Hawkins, WD Lust, et al. Baltimore, MD: Williams & Wilkins, 1980, p. 234–242.

Cahill Jr., GF, RL Veech. Ketoacids? Good medicine? *Trans Amer Clin Climatol Assoc* Vol 114 (2003): 149–163.

Clarke K, K Tchabanenko, R Pawlosky, et al. Oral 28-day and developmental toxicity studies of (R)-3-hydroxybutyl (R)-3-hydroxybutyrate. *Regulatory Toxicology and Pharmacology* Vol. 63 (2012): 196–208.

Cunnane S, S Nugent, M Roy, et al. Brain fuel metabolism, aging, and Alzheimer's disease. *Nutrition* Vol 27, No 1 (2011): 3–20.

Hasselbalch SG, PL Madsen, LP Hageman, et al. Changes in cerebral blood flow and carbohydrate metabolism during acute hyperketonemia. *Amer J Physiol* Vol 270 (1996): E746–751.

Kashiwaya Y, C Bergman, J-H Lee, et al. A ketone ester diet exhibits anxiolytic and cognition-sparing properties, and lessens amyloid and tau pathologies in a mouse model of Alzheimer's. *Neurobiol Aging* Vol 34, No 6 (2013): 1530–1539.

Kashiwaya Y, K Sato, N Tsuchiya, et al. Control of glucose utilization in working perfused rat heart. *J Biol Chem* Vol 269, No 41 (1994): 25502–25514.

Kashiwaya Y, T Takeshima, N Mori, et al. D-b-hydroxybutyrate protects neurons in models of Alzheimer's and Parkinson's disease. *PNAS* Vol 97, No 10 (2000): 5440–5444.

Kossoff EH, Zupec-Kania BA, Amark PE, et al. Optimal clinical management of children receiving the ketogenic diet: recommendations of the international ketogenic diet study group. *Epilepsia* Vol 50, No 2 (2009): 304–317.

Newport MT, TB VanItallie, Y Kashiwaya, et al. A new way to produce hyperketonemia: Use of ketone ester in a case of Alzheimer's disease. *Alzheimer's & Dementia* Vol. 11, No. 1 (2015): 99–103.

Owen OE, AP Morgan, GF Cahill Jr, et al. Brain metabolism during fasting. *J Clin Invest* Vol 46 (1967): 1589–1595.

Page KA, A Williamson, N Yu, et al. Medium-chain fatty acids improve cognitive function in intensively treated type 1 diabetic patients and support in vitro synaptic transmission during acute hypoglycemia. *Diabetes* Vol 58, No 5 (2009): 1237–1244.

Ridgel AL, JL Vitek, JL Alberts. Forced, not voluntary, exercise improves motor function in Parkinson's disease patients. *Neurorehabil Neural Repair* Vol 23, No 6 (2009): 600–608.

Seyfried TN, J Marsh, P Mukherjee, et al. Could metabolic therapy become a viable alternative to the standard of care for managing glioblastoma? *Hematology and Oncology Review* Vol 10, No 1 (2014): 13–20.

Srivastava S, Y Kashiwaya, MT King, et al. Mitochondrial biogenesis and increased uncoupling protein 1 in brown adipose tissue of mice fed a ketone ester diet. *FASEB J.* Vol 26, No 6 (2012): 2351–2362.

VanItallie TB, C Nonas, A Di Rocco, et al. Treatment of Parkinson disease with diet-induced hyperketonemia: a feasibility study. *Neurology* Vol 64 (2005): 728–730.

VanItallie TB, TH Nufert. Ketones: metabolism's ugly duckling. *Nutr Rev* Vol 61, No 10 (2003): 327–341.

Veech RL. The therapeutic implications of ketone bodies: the effects of ketone bodies inpathological conditions: ketosis, ketogenic diet, redox states, insulin resistance, and mitochondrial metabolism. *Prostaglandins, Leukot Essent Fatty Acids* Vol 70 (2004): 309–319.

Veech RL, B Chance, Y Kashiwaya, et al. Hypothesis paper: ketone bodies, potential therapeutic uses. *IUBMB Life* Vol 51 (2001): 241–247.

Appendix 2

Alzheimer's Disease Information Network. Undiagnosed pre-diabetes highly prevalent in early Alzheimer's disease. *ADIN Monthly E-News* No 57 (Aug 2013): 1–2.

Carter C. Alzheimer's disease: APP, Gamma Secretase, APOE, CLU, CR1, PICALM, ABCA7, BIN1, CD2AP, CD33, EPHA1, andMS4A2, and their relationships with herpes simplex, *C. pneumoniae,* other suspect pathogens, and the immune system. *Internat J Alzheimer's Dis* Vol 2011 (2011): 1–34.

Fleminger S, DL Oliver, S Lovestone, et al. Head injury as a risk factor for Alzheimer's disease: The evidence ten years on; a partial replication. *J Neurol Neurosurg Psychiatry* Vol 74 (2003): 857–862.

Mortimer JA, CM Van Duijn, V Chandra, et al. Head trauma as a risk factor for Alzheimer's disease: a collaborative re-analysis of case-controlled studies. *Int J Epidemiol* Vol 20, Suppl 2 (1991): S28–35.

Nedergaard M. Garbage truck of the brain. *Science* Vol 340, No 6140 (2013): 1529–1530.

Schwarz A. Dementia risk seen in players in NFL study. *New York Times,* Sept 30, 2009.

Index

About the Author

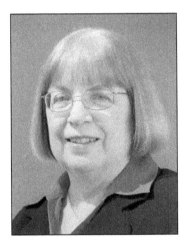

Mary T. Newport, M.D., grew up in Cincinnati, Ohio, and was educated at Xavier University and University of Cincinnati College of Medicine, both in Cincinnati. She is board certified in pediatrics and neonatology, and completed her training at Children's Hospital Medical Center in Cincinnati and at Medical University Hospital in Charleston, South Carolina. She has practiced in Florida since 1983 and was founding medical director of the newborn intensive care units at Mease Hospital Dunedin in 1987 and at Spring Hill Regional Hospital in 2002, where she practiced full-time until mid-2013. In mid-2014, Dr. Newport embarked on a new direction in medical practice at the opposite end of the spectrum, providing home visits to people who are homebound or receiving end-of-life care, which naturally grew out of her interest in Alzheimer's disease. She is a volunteer clinical assistant professor at the University of South Florida.

Dr. Newport is also the primary caregiver for her husband of forty-two years, Steve, who suffers from early-onset Alzheimer's disease. Her first book *Alzheimer's Disease: What If There Was a*

Cure? The Story of Ketones, now in its second edition, has been translated into French, German, Japanese, and several other languages. Dr. Newport has presented on this subject at the Alzheimer's Disease International Conferences in Thessaloniki, Greece, in 2010, and at many medical and nutrition-related conferences in North America, Europe, and Asia, and in 2013 gave a talk for TEDx. She also frequently appears on radio programs, podcasts, and television. Dr. Newport maintains a website, blog, and Facebook page to provide information about ketones as alternative fuel for the brain and the use of coconut and MCT oils in the diet at www.coconutketones.com and www.facebook.com/CoconutOil andAlzheimers.